BASIC SURGICAL TECHNIQUES

SIXTH EDITION

R.M. Kirk, MS FRCS

Honorary Professor of Surgery, University College London Medical School;

Honorary Consulting Surgeon, The Royal Free Hospital, London, UK

CHURCHILL LIVINGSTONE

ELSEVIER

Edinburgh   London   New York   Oxford   Philadelphia   St Louis   Sydney   Toronto 2010

CHURCHILL LIVINGSTONE

First published 1973
Second edition 1978
Third edition 1989
Fourth edition 1994
Fifth edition 2002
Sixth edition 2010

ISBN 978-0-7020-3391-9
  Reprinted 2010, 2012, 2013, 2014 (twice), 2015, 2016
International ISBN 978-0-7020-3390-2
  Reprinted 2011, 2012, 2014 (twice), 2015, 2016

British Library Cataloguing in Publication Data
A catalogue record for this book is available from the British Library

Library of Congress Cataloging in Publication Data
A catalog record for this book is available from the Library of Congress

---

Notice

Knowledge and best practice in this field are constantly changing. As new research and experience broaden our knowledge, changes in practice, treatment and drug therapy may become necessary or appropriate. Readers are advised to check the most current information provided (i) on procedures featured or (ii) by the manufacturer of each product to be administered, to verify the recommended dose or formula, the method and duration of administration, and contraindications. It is the responsibility of the practitioner, relying on their own experience and knowledge of the patient, to make diagnoses, to determine dosages and the best treatment for each individual patient, and to take all appropriate safety precautions. To the fullest extent of the law, neither the Publisher nor the Author assumes any liability for any injury and/or damage to persons or property arising out of or related to any use of the material contained in this book.

The Publisher

Printed in China

Working together to grow
libraries in developing countries

www.elsevier.com | www.bookaid.org | www.sabre.org

ELSEVIER **BOOK AID International** **Sabre Foundation**

The Publisher's policy is to use **paper manufactured from sustainable forests**

BASIC
SURGICAL
TECHNIQUES

For my grandchildren

Senior Commissioning Editor: Laurence Hunter
Development Editor: Sally Davies
Project Manager: Elouise Ball
Designer: Charles Gray
Illustration Manager: Bruce Hogarth
Illustrator: Antbits

Preface

Not everything that counts can be counted, and not everything that can be counted counts.
(Sign on Albert Einstein's study wall at Princeton University)

This is a 'How to do it' book. 'What to do' is described in surgical texts such as *General Surgical Operations* and *Essential General Surgical Operations*, both also published by Elsevier Churchill Livingstone. I have spent my whole career working with, and observing, masters and trainees in all branches of surgery. They all have their individual techniques but one aim in common – the safe, effective performance of operations on fellow humans.

Before the middle of the 19th century, surgeons were forced to operate on unanaesthetized patients as swiftly as possible. In Boston, Massachusetts, William Morton demonstrated the use of ether in 1846 and Sir James Young Simpson used chloroform in 1847. Now surgeons could work more gently and deliberately. Three giants and friends, Theodore Kocher in Berne, William Halsted in Baltimore and Harvey Cushing in New Hampshire, laid down the precepts of good operative skill. Techniques, instruments and materials have subsequently changed, but the correct method of handling living, healthy or diseased, human tissues has not. That is the subject of this book.

Success in surgery is not achieved just in the operating theatre; excellent decision-making, planning and preparation are undermined unless the operation is competently performed. Surgery (G *cheir* = hand + *ergon* = work; manual work), is a craft procedure. Craftsmen are expert at manipulating (L *manus* = hand + *plere* = to fill) a specific material, such as wood, leather, textiles and glass, and develop intimate knowledge on how to control them. We must learn to control our 'material', the living flesh of our patients; hence each chapter heading incorporates 'Handling …'.

How do you acquire exceptional skill? Much as I should like to claim it, this book cannot transmit surgical skill, neither can skills courses. As a former deviser and teacher of skills courses I am aware that they are a valuable introduction to – but not a replacement of – operative experience under expert guidance. They set basic standards of safe procedural practice and handling of instruments and equipment. They cannot show how to handle the target of the instruments, which is the patient's body, for which we have yet to produce simulations with the necessary complex, varied characteristics and texture.

A skill is so much more than a knowing. Great craftsmen, artists, actors, sportsmen, musicians may have inborn talent but they have applied it with enormous concentration, effort and single-minded purpose to reach the heights. Many, at the pinnacle of their success, nevertheless engage trainers and coaches to encourage, focus and correct their performance. Few of us have the potential but all of us who wish to apply ourselves to the highest achievable level need to recognize the complex mix of components required, and have the determination to achieve the best standard that we can.

To become a surgeon you need to fulfil certain training criteria and pass a number of examinations and assessments. Modern demands for objectivity determine the inclusion of tests that can be answered 'Yes' or 'No', awarded a statistically justifiable mark or produce a list. Thus the examiners influence the curriculum by including only what can be examined, not the whole of what is important. Questions that can be answered objectively are 'black' or 'white', whereas most of the questions of importance are various shades of grey – and are subjective. Lists beguile you into giving equal importance to each entry – nearly always, some are important, others are 'makeweight'. You may be capable of passing the examinations, but do not delude yourself into claiming that this success alone makes you a skilful surgeon.

Previous generations of surgeons learned their craft by watching, assisting and copying master surgeons. A teacher, or trainer, who may or may not be a surgeon, can transmit facts, describe procedures and assess their performance – but does not necessarily have the personal skill to demonstrate the procedures to the highest standards. A true master teaches by example. Do not despise the opportunity to watch and assist experts! The polymath Michael Polanyi (in *Personal Knowledge: Towards a Post-critical Philosophy*, Routledge & Kegan Paul, 1973) stated, 'By watching the master and emulating his efforts in the presence of his example, the apprentice unconsciously picks up the rules of the art, including those which are not explicitly known to the master himself.'

No one reads textbooks like this from cover to cover, so I do not feel guilty for repeating important statements, explanations and warnings.

Note

Many people whose first language is not English learn and practise surgery using English. When we learn surgery we encounter new words and usually assume the meaning from the context, but this is not always correct. The English language is a rich mixture of the Germanic (approximately 30%), Romance (approximately 60%), and is further enriched by additions from the languages of all the countries with which we have had contact.

I did not have the good fortune to be educated classically. How I regret that no-one explained the new vocabulary I encountered as a medical student. I learned words like 'parotid', unaware that it is Greek *para* = beside + *otis* = ear. I was recently entranced to read that 'parenchyma', which I should have found difficult to define accurately, was introduced by Erasistratus of the Alexandrian school about 300 BC, who thought that the organs were poured in from the blood and congealed (G *enchain* = to pour in). I make no apology for giving the origins and meanings of interesting words and mentioning contributors to surgical knowledge. Start your own voyage of discovery. You have entered a wonderful, historic profession and I hope you will enjoy reading of some of the words and people associated with it.

Word origins: G = Greek, L = Latin, LL = Low (or Late) Latin, Ger = German, OE = Old English, F = French.

Apologies

Once more I apologize to women surgeons if I have inadvertently written of 'he' and 'his' instead of 'he and she' and 'his and hers.' Since there is no epicene word for he and she, there are occasions when it is clumsy to keep repeating them. Secondly, the word 'master' in the connotation of expert, could not be accompanied with 'mistress', which has quite another meaning!

I have tried in this edition to take into account left-handed surgeons by referring where possible to 'dominant' and 'non-dominant' hand.

R.M. Kirk
London, 2010

Acknowledgements

This is a 'one man' production. Because I wished to demonstrate that skills are transferable, I did not wish to make it a multi-author text. However, I have a number of distinguished colleagues, with specialized knowledge, who have generously read through chapters, advised, inspired me, and corrected me, to whom I wish to pay tribute. Any remaining inaccuracies are mine.

Past and present colleagues at the Royal Free Hospital and in the UK

Mr Michael Brough, who sadly died prematurely; Miss Glenda Baillie, Mr Daryll Baker, Mr Jack Bradley, Mr Richard Brueton, Professor Peter Butler, Mr John Cochrane, Dr Michael Dashwood, Mr Peter Dawson, Professor Brian Davidson, Miss Linda de Cossart, Professor Amar Dhillon, Dr Robert Dick, Miss Deborah Eastwood, Professor George Hamilton, Mr Jonathan Jagger, Dr Simond Jaggernauth, Mr Mohammed Keshtgar, Professor Peter Lee, Mr Brian Little, Miss Bryony Lovett, Mr Alexander MacLeod, Mr Adam Magos, Professor Viswanath Mahadevan, Miss Ruth Manners, Professor Averil Mansfield, Matron Lesley Mattin SRN, Mr John Meyrick-Thomas, Mr Peter Mitchenere, Mr Richard Novell, Mr Olagunju Ogunbiyi, Mr Clive Quick, Mr Keith Rolles, Mr Geoffrey Sagor, Mr Paul Savage, Mr John Shaw, Mr William E. G. Thomas, Mr Christopher Uff, Mr Peter Veitch.

International colleagues

Professor Hiroshi Akiyama (Tokyo Japan), Professor Arjuna Aliwuhare (Peradinya, Sri Lanka), Professor Frantisek Antos (Prague, Czech Republic), Professor Sami Asfar (Kuwait), Mr Peter Cosman (Sydney, Australia), Professor Ken Cox (Sydney, Australia), Professor Waldemar Jedrzejczyk (Torun, Poland), Professor Samiran Nundy (Delhi, India), Professor Krishna Reddy (Chennai, India), Professor Adib Rizvi (Karachi, Pakistan), Professor Harushi Udagawa (Tokyo, Japan).

It is a pleasure to thank the editorial and production team at Elsevier: Laurence Hunter, Sally Davies, Charles Gray, Elouise Ball and Antbits.

Contents

Chapter | 1 |

Handling yourself

The personal qualities you bring to medicine are the same as those that drive all clinicians. We are all primarily physicians, endeavouring to apply the same knowledge and judgement that our medical colleagues apply to diagnosing and treating patients.

1. The extra, practical aptitude you must acquire beyond clinical competence is operating skill – the ability to manipulate living human tissue with intimate knowledge of its characteristics in health and disease, while endeavouring to preserve its physical and functional qualities. In the medieval period surgeons, unlike physicians, did not study at a university but were ranked as craftsmen, learning as apprentices from masters. As in other trades, surgeons use tools or instruments to facilitate controlling their materials but recognize that they are intermediates between their hands and the object of their skill. Your awareness of this should impress on you the need to use every practical task you perform as a means of improving the skills required in surgery – all day, every day, not just in the operating theatre.

2. Individual components of operative skill can be listed but do not define the way in which they are put together to create a successful surgeon. Few of us are fully equipped mentally and physically, but by putting in the extra effort to overcome our weaknesses, we hope to compensate for them. In contrast some, fortunate enough to be born with natural aptitudes fail to put in the extra effort.

3. In this chapter I hope to demonstrate how to identify in yourself some of the qualities you need to utilize and develop in order to become a skilful surgeon. You can recognize the presence or lack of them in your everyday life and initiate your training even before you step into the operating theatre. Continue this process when you watch operations, become an assistant, and are eventually allowed to perform part or all of an operation.

4. It is not necessary to see someone operating to identify the presence or absence of desirable qualities. Watch others performing everyday tasks such as carving a joint of meat, peeling fruit, eating a meal; is the food on the plate still orderly – or does it look like a battlefield? Note someone who habitually drops objects and swears at them muttering 'Bad luck. That happens every time.' Why do experts not suffer such misfortunes? They recognize the likelihood and incorporate precautionary measures into their routines.

5. Some accomplish everyday tasks calmly, safely, in an orderly manner, maintaining uncluttered surroundings. Others are casual, messy, rough, clumsy with their hands, the equipment, or the object which

they are handling, and do not seem to anticipate an imminent fault or accident that is evident to the onlookers. They may be outstanding at their vocation but you would feel anxious if they claimed to be surgeons or intended to pursue such a career.

ATTITUDES – THE FIVE 'Cs'

1. *Common sense* encompasses being aware at all times of what is going on around you and reacting to it in a logical and rational manner. It is eroded if you are distracted, lose your composure and temper, so your anticipation of impending danger is blunted, as is your ability to react sensibly and perform effectively. If you encounter a difficulty do not rush wildly into 'doing something'. Respond to changed circumstances; errors often result from dogged and blind continuation with the intended procedure; this is sometimes (but not by me) entitled 'situational awareness'.

2. *Competence.* Make it a habit in your everyday life to carry out your duties in a relaxed atmosphere of expertise and calm. List your intentions in descending order of priority and ensure you are able to carry them out proficiently and professionally. Take each step in its correct order, complete it, check it and continue with the next one – but react to new input and if necessary respond to it.

3. *Commitment.* Keep in mind your prime purpose. Unless circumstances change, concentrate on this and do not be deflected from it without good reason. Be willing to defer or cancel other duties in order to fulfil the most important one. Except in an emergency, complete every task.

4. *Compassion.* How privileged you are to be a physician, able to treat patients who are in pain, or anxious. Now you wish to add to your skills and offer another means of treatment. Operating on people can be dramatically successful – and also disastrous. Expect to have occasional sleepless nights from anxiety and guilt as you retrospectively consider your recent actions.

5. *Communication.* You are in a professional relationship with your patients, their relatives, and your colleagues. Technical skill in the operating theatre is not sufficient on its own to make you

a successful surgeon. It is a vital add-on but it is one component among many others. You must communicate and be open to communication – listen, as well as talk.

PHYSICAL ATTRIBUTES

Hands

1. There is no ideal surgeon's hand. The shape of your hand has little or no bearing on your manipulative skill. However, identify the peculiarities of your own hands and fingers in order to exploit the benefits and make the best use of them. For example, the terminal phalanx, nail shape and extent of nail bed towards the tips of your fingers affect your preference for fingertip pressure or pulp pressure.

2. Your hands are important assessors of tissues. Their sensitivity is affected by wearing gloves. When clinical circumstances require you to wear gloves, consciously note the changes. Make sure you wear the correct size of gloves and wear them correctly. Do not allow the glove fingertips to project beyond yours – pull the glove fingers on fully, if necessary creating concertina'd wrinkles near the base of your fingers.

3. There are many outstanding left-handed surgeons so this is no disability, even though many instruments are designed for right-handed people.

Stability

1. Surgeons do not usually have extraordinarily steady hands. Our ability to perform finely controlled movements diminishes as we age.

2. If you hold long-handled instruments at arm's length, the tips magnify the tremor – and anxiety exaggerates this. Do not feel embarrassed. The further the distance from a firm base to the point of action, the less steady are your hands.

3. Stand upright with feet apart, arms and fingers outstretched. You will detect a slight tremor at your outspread fingertips. Now press your elbows into your sides and you should find your hands are steadier. Sit, or brace your hips against a fixture to become even steadier. Rest your elbows on a table; also rest the heel of your hand or your little finger on the table (Fig. 1.1).

Key point

- Keep a firm base as close as possible to the point of action.

Fig. 1.1 Your wrist and little finger rest on the base, forming a steadying bridge while you hold the scalpel to make a precise incision.

Fig. 1.2 Steadying an instrument by resting it on the fingers of the other hand.

4. If you cannot use a base close to the active fingers, use the other hand to steady the dominant hand by grasping the wrist. If you need to reach to make an action – for example when you are cutting ligatures as an assistant, use the fingers of the inactive hand on which to rest the scissors (Fig. 1.2). If no other base exists, place the 'heels' of your hands together when carrying out a manoeuvre such as the nowadays rare need to thread a needle (Fig. 1.3).
5. If you need to carry out a smooth movement, try practising it in the air first, as a golfer does before making a stroke.

WHAT IS SKILL?

1. The Old Norse word 'skil' signified distinction (from *skilja* = to separate, discriminate). In everyday use it commonly signifies expertise and dexterity

Fig. 1.3 Press your wrists together while threading a needle.

in performing a practical procedure as opposed to facility in a theoretical or abstract accomplishment.
2. As an example, a tennis beginner must learn to control the racket to strike a ball. Initially the player must concentrate on the dominant hand controlling the racket head. As the presence of the racket becomes a familiar extension of the hand, the concentration can be transferred increasingly to the ball, which becomes the prime focus as its flight is observed and predicted. The racket head is relegated to subsidiary focus[1] and seems to move naturally so that the sweet spot impacts on the ball.
3. This ability to 'download' the means of accomplishing something, so freeing the performer to focus attention on the prime object of the procedure, is a skill. It is a fundamental achievement that has to be acquired by assiduous, intelligent practice. It frees the player to see the game as a whole, able to plan, anticipate and be correctly positioned for the next shot.
4. It is remarkable that having acquired a skill and then trying to add further ones, the first skill is initially lost. When you learn to drive a car, having learned to control the accelerator and brake, if you now look at the other traffic, as you wish to signal your desire to move off and steer into the road, your control of the accelerator and brake pedals often regresses.
5. When you have acquired a skill, however simple, you will find that if you concentrate on it, you become clumsy. If you are familiar with a QWERTY keyboard on a computer or typewriter, ask yourself if you can continue the line of letters after the 'Y' or list the next line. Why do you have difficulty? Your fingers go to them automatically because you have relegated them to a subsidiary awareness. Your focal awareness is directed at what you are writing.

6. You will appreciate that if you attempt to hurry, you are moving your primary focus from the accomplishment of the skilful performance to the individual movements, and you make mistakes. Take the example once again of the keyboard. Try typing at speed. Your focal awareness shifts to the keys, not to the content – and you make mistakes.

> **Key points**
>
> - Having acquired a skill, always perform it at a natural pace.
> - Hand speed and work speed are not parallel – they may even be opposed.
> - Indeed, it often takes longer to repeat and correct a rushed and imperfect act than to perform it deliberately and correctly in the first place.

7. In order to acquire a skill you must practise it assiduously until you can perform it repeatedly and reliably. Just going through movements does not demonstrate a skill. You need to perform it perfectly, every time.

8. Watch and copy experts. Of course, they cannot bestow skill. Differentiate between trainers and masters. A trainer or coach can tell you what to do, assess you and identify ways to improve but does not necessarily have the personal skill to do it at a high level. A craft master (L *magister*) is one who is expert at *performing* the craft – and can show you. Watch and remember how they achieve their success.

EXERCISES VERSUS PRACTICE

1. Since you need to carry out the task repeatedly to acquire skill, differentiate between exercise and practice. It is a distinction recognized more by instrumental musicians and those pursuing a career in sports, than by surgeons.

2. *Exercise.* If you wish to become accomplished at a particular procedure you have been shown, you may repeat it until it becomes second nature and you can carry it out without the need to concentrate on the component actions. Each repetition is the same as the previous one. The Suzuki method of teaching young violinists uses this method.

3. *Practice.* You may instead perform the manoeuvre, identify a difficulty or a means of facilitating it, adjust the next trial to judge its success in eliminating the difficulty, and making the procedure easier, better controlled and feeling more natural. Continue until you cannot improve it further and only then do you convert it into an exercise.[2]

4. Remain willing to modify it again if you find a better routine. One of the benefits of watching others is that it gives you the opportunity to see new approaches to difficult manoeuvres. Musical instrumentalists often ask experts to 'finger in' passages which they find difficult.

5. This intelligent practice augments the natural process of skills learning in which as we repeat a manoeuvre we develop a confidence in the probability of the next result and adjust the 'feed-forward' motor signals. During the performance, sensorimotor signals provide 'feed-back' adjustments to create the optimum result. This is a form of Bayesian integration.[3]

HAPTICS

1. Do not be distracted by this word (G *haptein* = to fasten). It is well known in industry but relatively new in medicine and surgery. It becomes increasingly important as we introduce methods of 'handling' tissues by instruments that reduce or remove our ability to feel them, assess their surface, texture, temperature, and appreciate the force we are applying to them and their resistance to that force. It is the science of touch (possibly related to L *tangere* = to touch), creating an interface mainly between us and technological apparatus and instruments.[4]

2. During clinical examination of our patients we recognize and identify many structures by touch, assessing the surface, texture and temperature. We employ our kinaesthetic sense (G *kinein* = to move + *aisthesis* = perception) to explore them for homogeneity, strength, friability, flexibility and attachments. We may receive force feedback from resistance or vibrations. We rely heavily on our knowledge of the texture of structures and when we wear gloves, even thin surgical gloves, our appreciation of touch is impaired.

3. When you interpose an instrument between your hand and the target structure your tactile input is drastically reduced. Rigid instruments such as dissecting forceps, transmit more than do soft or flexible ones; when you pass a soft urinary catheter into the bladder you need to move it extremely delicately to appreciate the progress through the urethra. The more complex the link between hand and target structure, the greater the loss of touch.

4. You will find, as you embark on your surgical career that much of your training will be using instruments. Do not be misled into feeling that skill in manipulating them alone confers surgical skill. However, many surgical procedures are now performed without the operator touching the tissues. In order to reduce the exposure, minimal access procedures have been widely developed. When using

instruments, whether hand-held, mechanically or electronically linked, the sense of touch is reduced or lost. You may have the opportunity to experience on a simulator, the use of minimal access instruments, often with relatively long handles and the need to move your hand in the opposite direction to the intended tip movement. In robotic surgery the hand and target tissue are decoupled, being driven through electronic systems. Much research is directed at providing force feedback to the operator to help in the estimation of the tissues held within graspers.[5]

5. *Force and torque.* In other occupations artificially produced haptic feedback systems are in use to provide operators with, as yet limited, sensation of feel and measure of applied force and torque (L *torquere* = to twist). These are being introduced into surgical applications. When you watch an expert tighten a ligature it is impossible to know, and accurately replicate, the tension. Again, in the case of hand-held or electronically controlled robotic instruments, appreciation of the force transmitted is reduced or not sensed. It is now possible to measure the force exerted through some instruments.[6] An important finding is that novices tend to exert up to 130% more force or torque than is required by experts to perform the same procedure.

You do not need elaborate equipment to recognize the potential damage you can inadvertently create by pinching tissues with instruments. If the handles of hinged forceps are twice as long as the blades, your squeezing force is doubled at the tips. You may exert very high compression per unit area through fine forceps with tip surfaces as fine as 2–3 mm². Use too much force and when you release your pressure the crushed tissue soon looks normal – but it will die or at best be partially replaced with scar. When you look at some old wounds, you see scarred lines crossing the healed wound – they result from too tightly tied sutures.

Whenever you encounter resistance, of any type, make it a habit to apply the minimum force to overcome it. Often this means changing your approach, method, or removing an obstacle that adds to the difficulty. When you watch or assist an expert surgeon you will be surprised how little force is used. Magically, the tissues seem to behave well out of respect for the surgeon. It is not magic. It is the result of intimate familiarity in guiding the tissues to conform to the operator's wishes. This is the essence of craftsmanship.

Key points

- Make it a habit in everyday activities, to achieve manipulations with minimal force.
- Consider trying several methods and choose the gentlest.

TRANSFERABLE SKILLS

1. Even before you enter the operating theatre you can start to develop or improve the manipulative facility and sensitivity that you will require as a surgeon. Adapt every possible normal routine to hone your skills. Watch skilled workers in other vocations and you will see common traits, some of which you can incorporate into your training. It is a joy to see someone carefully assessing a problem, unhurriedly preparing the materials and tools, doing the preparatory work to facilitate the task, now seemingly effortlessly carrying out the needed procedure, reassembling, testing and approving the result. This is a demonstration of seamless assessment, decision, preparation, accomplishment, final assessment without haste or the need to correct imperfections.

2. The French surgeon Alexis Carrel (1873–1944) developed his suturing technique after watching an expert embroiderer in Lyon. He practised by inserting up to 500 stitches in a cigarette paper without once tearing it, becoming a founder of vascular surgery, for which he received the Nobel Prize in 1912. The British surgeon Lord Moynihan (1865–1936), who was famously skilled, was reported to carry a piece of string with which he practised tying knots whenever he had a spare moment.

3. As examples, when you peel a fruit, or open a sealed envelope, you can practise separating tissues without damaging them, while keeping in the correct plane. You achieve this by keeping the distance between the adherent surfaces and the distracting force to a minimum. Every time you open a sealed envelope, raise an edge of the flap and extend the parting. Grasp each edge between thumb and index finger. While keeping your index fingers pressed together, evert your hands so that the edges are separated. Limit the extent of the cleaving tension by compressing the still sealed section just ahead of the split between your middle fingers (Fig. 1.4). You are remarkably sensitive to incipient tearing. Unless you readjust your grip every few millimetres, your hands move apart, the extent of paper at risk is lengthened and you may not detect a tear starting anywhere along it.

4. Use your ingenuity to find other practice opportunities. Try to perform every action gently, neatly and with minimum disturbance.

Speed

The examples of focal awareness demonstrate the importance of allowing your hard-won skill to be applied naturally. Do not compromise the benefits of this by hurrying.

Fig. 1.4 Peeling apart two adherent strips. Trap the strips between the thumbs and index fingers. As you supinate your wrists, you separate the strips but maintain contact between your index fingers and then your middle fingers. This keeps the length of strips being distracted to a minimum. Do not separate your hands but repeatedly change your grip.

Sequence (L *sequi* = to follow)

If you need to take apart, adjust and repair any structure or equipment, determine to attempt it without misplacing or dropping any part, and carry out the dismantling and re-assembly in the correct sequence. The value of the habit will be evident when you watch or participate in a surgical operation. There is a well-tried procedural order.

SKILLS COURSES

1. In the past trainee surgeons watched, assisted and then operated on patients. Indeed there was an adage, 'See one, do one, teach one.' It is preferable for you to be shown in a course, away from the potentially tense atmosphere of an operating theatre, how to perform the procedures and carry them out under supervision and guidance. Take every opportunity to attend such courses.

2. Practice operations on live but anaesthetized animals is strictly limited except for microsurgery. For many years dead animal tissue has been used but increasingly, because of public health fears of transmitting viral and other infections, simulated tissues are used. The available models may look like the real body parts but it is not yet possible to create simulations with the complex, varied structure and consistency that you will encounter in surgical practice. This is a serious deficiency. The ultimate purpose of these courses is to teach you to operate on living tissue, yet this is lacking.

3. You must become familiar with handling surgical instruments and courses offer you this facility. You initially need to concentrate your attention on controlling them, rather than controlling what is at the other end of them. As you become more familiar they become natural extensions of your hand and when you come to operate on living tissues, you can focus your concentration on the tissues rather than on the instruments, with which you are now proficient (see below).

4. Minimal access surgical courses are particularly valuable because you need to become familiar with the opposite effects of hand movements on instrument tip movement through the pivoted access port (see Ch. 13).

5. Virtual reality instruments and courses based on them provide you with the opportunity to learn how to control complex instruments that further remove you from the target tissues. At present they mainly offer exercises that you control under visual guidance. They offer the promise of greater haptic and force/torque feedback (see above).

> ### Key points
>
> - Skills courses offer excellent introductions to operative procedures. They are adjuncts, not replacements, for training on living tissues.
> - Skills courses do not transfer skills to you; they should reveal to you what skills you need to acquire by active practice.

6. *Create your own simulations.* Courses offer you a limited experience of carrying out operations. You need to create opportunities for practising the routines and become familiar with them. Use your ingenuity to create an arrangement that allows you to repeatedly follow through part or all of an operation. When you are offered the opportunity to carry out the same procedure in the operating theatre you will have the confidence to perform it competently. In the future, the surgeon, who is responsible to the patient, will be more willing to delegate a procedure to you if you have already demonstrated on a simulation that you can perform it safely.[7,8]

RATIONAL ASSESSMENT OF INFORMATION

1. Part of your complex development as a competent surgeon is how you discriminate the information you receive. You will be simultaneously trying to improve as a physician-scientist, a practical craftsman, learning current accepted practice, yet being aware that this may be rapidly changing.

2. Be willing to follow the practice of your teachers. This often means that you have to change your methods as you pass through the rotating appointments. It is important that you do not become too rigid early in your career. Sometimes an unfamiliar method proves, with practice, to be an improvement on your current one.
3. Your trainers may claim that their success depends upon some possibly unique change in their technique or material, yet they seem to get similar results to others who do not perform in the same manner. You will learn that it is not the method or the material that is the component of success but rather the care with which it is incorporated into the procedure. Your teacher is too modest in attributing success

to one change, when it is the result of outstanding commitment to skill and competence.

4. Improvements in techniques, instruments and materials constantly appear. Welcome them but assess them critically. Those who introduce them often unconsciously or consciously select the patients, and by committing to it greater effort and enthusiasm, obtain improved outcomes. Improvement in performance may also result from increased attention to it. This is often called the 'Hawthorne effect', named after a noted rise in productivity at a factory in Hawthorne near Chicago when the workers became aware that they were being assessed. It is only when uncommitted researchers detect improvement that you should embrace the claimed improvement.

REFERENCES

1. Polanyi M. *Personal knowledge*. London: Routledge & Kegan Paul; 1973.
2. Cross KD. Role of practice in perpetual-motor learning. *Am J Phys Med*. 1967;46:487–510.
3. Kording KP, Wolpert DM. Bayesian integration in sensorimotor learning. *Nature*. 2004;427:244–247.
4. Robles-de-La-Torre G. Principles of haptic perception in virtual environments. In: Grunwald M, ed. *Human haptic perception*. Birkhäuser Verlag: Basel; 2008:363–379.
5. Hannaford B, Trujillo J, Sinanan M, et al. Computerized surgical grasper. In: *Proceedings of Medicine Meets Virtual Reality*, pp. 55–57. San Diego, CA; 1998.
6. Rosen J, MacFarlane M, Richards C, et al. Surgeon-tool force/torque signatures: evaluation of surgical skills in minimally invasive surgery. In: *Proceedings of Medicine Meets Virtual Reality, MMVR – 7*, San Francisco, CA; IOS Press; 1999. Online. Available: http://bionics.soe.ucsc.edu/publications/CP_03.pdf June 26, 2009.
7. Kirk RM. Surgical skills and lessons from other vocations. *Ann R Coll Surg Engl*. 2006;88:95–98.
8. Beard JD, Jolly BC, Newble BI, et al. Assessing the technical skills of surgical trainees. *Br J Surg*. 2005;92:778–782.

FURTHER READING

Cosman P, Hemli JM, Ellis AM, Hugh TJ. Learning the surgical craft: a review of skills training options. *Aust N Z J Surg*. 2009;77:838–845.

Kirk RM. Teaching the craft of operative surgery. *Ann R Coll Surg Engl*. 1996;78:25–28.

Kirk RM. Surgical excellence – threats and opportunities. *Ann R Coll Surg Engl*. 1998;80:256–259.

Thomas WEG. Teaching and assessing surgical competence. *Ann R Coll Surg Engl*. 2006;88:429–432.

Chapter | 2 |

Handling instruments

Key points

- Do not delude yourself into thinking you are expert because you can handle instruments.
- Your expertise is measured ultimately by how you deal with the tissues.
- But familiarity with instruments frees you to concentrate on the living tissues.
- *You are ultimately responsible for the instrument count.*
- Make sure you retrieve them all before closing.

Learn to handle and become familiar with standard instruments, since they are surgical extensions of your hands. Practise using instruments that are employed in open surgery to carry out functions that you would expect to carry out in surgical procedures. Acquaint yourself with minimal access instruments using simple simulations (see Ch. 13) and for both these and endoscopes attend courses and practise on any available virtual reality instruments.

SCALPEL

The scalpel (L *scalpere* = to cut) is the traditional instrument of surgeons. Solid reusable knives are still used for cutting tough tissues, but some instruments are totally disposable.

If you use a scalpel with a disposable blade, fit and remove the blade while holding it clear of the sharp edge with forceps or needle-holder, not with fingers. If it slips you will avoid sustaining a cut.

1. Use a scalpel for making deliberate cuts into tissues, dividing them with the minimum trauma in order to cut skin, separate tissues to reach a targeted area, divide and resect tissues.
2. Draw the belly of the blade across the target rather than exerting excessive pressure that may result in an uncontrolled cut. Draw the knife blade under controlled pressure to determine the depth of cut.

Fig. 2.1 Hold the scalpel for making a long smooth incision. Draw the belly of the knife, not the point, from your non-dominant to you dominant side. If you are cutting along a sagittal plane, cut from far to near.

3. For cutting skin and similar structures, hold the knife in a manner similar to that for holding a table knife (Fig. 2.1). Keep the knife horizontal, suspended below your pronated hand, held between thumb and middle finger. Place your index finger on the back of the knife at the base of the blade, to control the pressure exerted on it. Wrap your ring and little fingers around the handle to reinforce your steadying grip, so that the end of the handle rests against the hypothenar eminence.

4. When you need to produce a small puncture, a short, precise incision, or cut a fine structure, hold the knife like a pen (see Fig. 1.1).

5. As a rule you cut in the sagittal plane (L *sagitta* = arrow; the path of an arrow directly away from you), from far to near, and in the transverse plane from non-dominant to dominant side. If you need to cut from dominant to non-dominant side, consider going to the other side of the operating table, using your non-dominant hand, or using scissors.

6. Do not misuse the scalpel by attempting to cut metal or bone, or try to lever the knife during a cutting manoeuvre. Do not continue to use a blunt scalpel, since once the sharp edge is lost, you need to apply excessive pressure and the incision is uneven.

7. Never make a casual incision without first assessing the exact situation; some are irretrievable. Before making a critical incision plan it and if necessary first draw an intended line on the skin with Bonney's blue ink. Occasionally it is worth practising in the air before making a smooth, controlled cut, as golfers do when preparing to make a putt. If an important structure will be endangered, interpose a protective instrument such as a retractor. When you are about to cut a linear structure in the depths you may be able to place a grooved dissector beneath it, to protect deeper tissues.

8. A special scalpel exists, called a bistoury, conjectured to be named after Pistorium (modern Pistoja) in Tuscany where they were made. It has a long thin curved blade, blunt-ended for side cutting, sharp tipped for end cutting through a small opening. I have never used one, preferring to improve the access and cut under direct vision.

SCISSORS

The cutting action of scissors (LL *cisorium* = a cutting instrument, from *caedere* = to cut) results from the moving edge contact between the blades, which are given a slight set towards each other. If you hold them up to the light, edge on, you should see light between the blades except at the joint and at one point of contact which moves towards the tips as you close the blades. If the blades spring apart the cutting action is replaced by a chewing effect and this results if delicate scissors are used to cut tough tissues.

Scissors are made for right-handed users and the lateral pressure of the right-handed thumb tends to result in the blades being pressed together. When held in the left hand the pressure of the thumb tends to lever the blades apart.

Most surgical scissors have round tips but for special purposes pointed blades may be used. The blades may be straight, curved or angled.

1. With your hand in mid-pronation, hold scissors by inserting only part of the first phalanx of the thumb through one ring (called a 'bow' by the manufacturers); this controls the moving blade. Insert only the first phalanx of the ring finger into the other ring, and wrap the middle and little fingers around the handle to steady it; this will be the fixed blade (Fig. 2.2). Place the tip of your index finger on the hinge.

2. If you are left-handed, using scissors to make a crucial cut, insert the whole terminal phalanx of your thumb through its ring so you can flex it at the interphalangeal joint and draw the ring to your left to increase the binding force between the blades.

3. As a rule your hand is most comfortable in the mid-prone position but if you are cutting down a deep hole try fully supinating your hand so that you have a clearer view of the structures at the tip. The knuckles of a hand in pronation may obstruct your view.

4. Choose the correct scissors for the task. Mayo's are excellent rounded tipped all-purpose scissors (from the celebrated Clinic of the brothers William born 1861, Charles born 1865, both died 1939, came well-designed scissors and needle-holder). Use lighter scissors for very light work only. Remember that it is more difficult to make curved scissors' blades accurately engage along their whole length. If you are cutting down a hole prefer long-handled scissors

Fig. 2.3 Cut from left to right while holding the scissors in your right hand.

Fig. 2.2 Insert only half the distal phalanx of your thumb, and all the distal phalanx of your ring finger through the rings of scissors. Wrap your middle and little fingers around the ring finger. Place your index finger on the hinge.

so that the rings remain outside the hole. The longer the scissors, the more likely is any tremor magnified, so be willing to rest the hinge on the fingers of your non-dominant hand (see Fig. 1.2).

5. It is fortunate that scalpel and scissors cut in opposite directions. Scissors cut in the sagittal plane from near to far but when you need to cut from far to near, it may be practical to use a scalpel. In the transverse plane scissors cut most conveniently from dominant towards the non-dominant side. When you need to cut in the transverse plane from your non-dominant side towards your dominant side, consider moving to the other side of the operating table or using a scalpel. If you are reasonably ambidextrous change the scissors to your non-dominant hand; alternatively swing the scissors round in your dominant hand, so they point towards your elbow (Fig. 2.3).

6. For rather snobbish reasons scissors are despised as a dissecting instrument by some, who consider that tissues should never be divided except with a scalpel. I must admit that some surgeons are a delight to watch, wielding a scalpel with great skill and effectiveness. However, appearance is not all. I have also admired surgeons using scissors with great versatility, inserting the tips into a tissue plane, gently

opening the blades to create a defined bridge of tissue, withdrawing the scissors, inserting one blade beneath, one blade superficial to the bridge and dividing it, proceeding in a rapid, effective manner, without the need to change instruments. Watch others, try both methods, make up your own mind. I suspect that you will conclude, like me, that there is room for both techniques.

Key point

- Invariably keep and pass sharp instruments in kidney dishes to avoid the risks of acquiring, or passing on, infection including viral diseases.

DISSECTING FORCEPS (THUMB FORCEPS)

It is not clear whether the word derived from *ferriceps* (L *ferrum* = iron + *capere* = to take) or from *formus* (L = hot + *capere*). They grip when compressed between thumb and fingers. When released the blades separate because they are made of springy steel. Dissecting forceps form an excellent multipurpose instrument. The commonest types are toothed and non-toothed but various shaped tips are available, such as rings for grasping soft viscera. Delicate forceps have a post on the inside of one blade that engages with a hole in the other blade, to ensure that the tips meet accurately. If you compress the forceps tightly the sharp post will protrude through the opposite blade and potentially pierce your glove or your skin – a sure sign that you are crushing the tissue between the blade tips. Dissecting forceps may be extremely delicate for use during microsurgery or large and strong for grasping tough tissues.

Toothed forceps have at least one tooth on one tip, interdigitating with two teeth on the opposing tip. The intention is that the teeth puncture the surface of the tissue, tethering it and so preventing it from slipping, rather than holding it by strong compression, which may be more damaging. Skin is tolerant of punctures but is severely injured by crushing, so toothed forceps are usually employed to grasp it. Very tough slippery tissues such as fascia, fibrocartilage and bone are best grasped with toothed forceps.

Non-toothed forceps exert their grip through serrations on the opposing surfaces. Use them when manipulating blood vessels, bowel and small ducts, since punctures of these cause leakage. Provided the closed tips are used to act as counter pressure and manipulate tissue rather than to grip it, they are suitable for use on skin, but skin hooks are preferable (see Ch. 6).

> ### Key points
>
> - The pressure exerted per unit area when fine-tipped forceps are forcibly closed is extremely high.
> - Tissues crushed by this force will appear normal soon afterwards – but will die.
> - Whenever possible use the closed tips to stabilize or distort tissues and create counter pressure.

1. As a rule hold dissecting forceps like a pen in your non-dominant hand, since you usually have another instrument in your dominant hand (Fig. 2.4). They do not usually have a locking mechanism because they are intended to provide only a temporary grip.
2. Learn to palm forceps (Fig. 2.5), retaining them with your ring and little fingers, to free the index and middle fingers, and thumb, while tying knots.
3. The closed blades of round-nosed non-toothed forceps make an excellent dissecting tool to open up a longitudinal tissue plane. Gently insert them in the desired plane as a wedge, and allow their springiness to open up and create a space between the

Fig. 2.4 Grip dissecting forceps like a pen but usually in your non-dominant hand, since you usually hold a scalpel or scissors in your dominant hand while dissecting.

Fig. 2.5 If you palm dissecting forceps, hold them with your ring and little fingers, freeing your important fingers to hold other instruments or tissues, or to tie knots.

blades along which you can identify and selectively divide the overlying tissue (see Ch. 9). This method is valuable when displaying a longitudinal structure such as a blood vessel, nerve or tendon.

ARTERY FORCEPS (HAEMOSTATIC FORCEPS, HAEMOSTATS)

Haemostatic forceps (G *haema* = blood + *stasis* = stoppage) were devised by the great French surgeon Ambroise Paré (1510–1590) with a scissors action, and were improved by the addition of a ratchet so they can be locked, by Sir Thomas Spencer Wells (1818–1897) after whom they are often named. Note that the tips alone meet when they are lightly closed; the proximal parts of the blades are slightly separated. The basic design is so versatile that it has been adapted from fine 'mosquito' forceps to heavy, toothed grasping forceps. Some haemostats are straight but most are curved.

1. Insert the first phalanx only of your thumb and of your ring finger into the rings of the opened forceps, with your index finger on the hinge. When the handles are compressed, the ratchets lock. To release them you need to compress them lightly to overcome the slight overhang of the ratchet, separate the handles in a plane at right angles to the hinge action, and open the handles. Practise the action so that you can skilfully and controllably apply and remove them automatically. As an assistant learn to use your non-dominant hand because you usually have scissors in your dominant hand, ready to cut the ligature.
2. Because these forceps can be applied and left in place, always ensure the shafts are sufficiently long so that the handles remain outside the wound.

Fig. 2.7 Learn to remove artery forceps with your non-dominant hand in a controlled manner, without allowing them to spring off. As an assistant you normally hold your scissors in your dominant hand, ready to cut the ends of the ligature to the correct length.

Fig. 2.6 When applying curved haemostatic forceps to capture bleeding vessels, prefer to have your hand supinated, and with curved forceps, have the convexity down, and ensure the tips just project beyond the vessel.

Short-handled forceps left in the wound are easily forgotten, so always check the number at the end of the procedure.

3. Apply artery forceps to bleeding vessels with your hand supinated, the convexity of curved forceps facing down (Fig. 2.6). Grasp vessels so the tips of the forceps protrude; this retains the subsequently applied ligature, preventing it from slipping over the tip and trapping the forceps in the tied ligature. If this happens, when the forceps are removed, they will pull off the ligature. A single click of the ratchet may suffice.

4. Avoid picking up extraneous tissue. If you apply a ligature around it and the vessel, the attachment will anchor the ligature and allow the vessel, as it retracts, to withdraw from it and rebleed.

5. If you are the assistant, you will be expected to remove the forceps when the vessel is ligated. The surgeon will either expect you to lift the handle of the forceps to allow the end of the ligature to be passed from hand to hand on your side of the vessel, or will stretch the ligature between two hands on your side of the vessel while you reach over it to grasp the handles of the forceps. As the first half-hitch is formed and tightened, you should, when requested, release and remove the haemostat in a controlled manner. If you leave the forceps, they may prevent the first half-hitch from being tightened. Grasp the far ring between your index finger and thumb; this is to be the static ring. Insert part of the first phalanx of the ring finger in the other ring and steady it by pressure from outside

the ring, with the little finger (Fig. 2.7). Gently compress the rings together to release the overlap of the ratchet, lever the handles in opposite directions at right angles to the joint and gently open the forceps without pulling them off. When the final half-hitch has been tightened the surgeon will hold up the ends of the ligature while you cut them, using the scissors held in the right hand. When an important vessel is being tied you may be asked to slacken the forceps while a first ligature is being tied and tightened; then re-clamp the forceps while a second ligature is tied and tightened, before removing the forceps.

TISSUE FORCEPS

These rely for their grip on the shape and apposing surfaces of their blades in contact with the tissues to grasp but not damage them. Some encircle the tissues, some have large ring blades through which the tissues bulge, or rough surfaces, or teeth (Fig. 2.8).

1. Use them in circumstances when traction sutures or a sharp hook may cut out, when the tissues are too slippery to be held with smooth retractors, and when the direction of traction needs to be varied. Do not use metal forceps when gravity, tapes, packing, or extending the incision could be less damaging.

2. If you need to apply strong traction of tough tissues, use forceps with a powerful grip rather than inadequate forceps that are likely to pull off, tearing the tissues and straining the forceps. When the tissues are fragile, use delicate forceps, apply them carefully, do not drag on them and remove them as soon as possible. Several lightweight forceps may give a better grip and do less damage than a single pair of heavy forceps.

Fig. 2.8 Tissue-holding forceps. **A** Allis. **B** Lane's. **C** Ring.
D Babcock's. **E** Duval. **F** Kocher's.

Fig. 2.9 Needle-holders. **A** Mayo's. **B** Gillies' incorporating scissors. **C** One type of ophthalmic needle-holder.

NEEDLE-HOLDERS

In the past we frequently held needles in our hands. The risk of sustaining or transmitting infection, especially viral and prion diseases, has made the practice unsustainable. There is a great variety of needle-holders but relatively few are in common use (Fig. 2.9). They grip the needle with specially designed jaws. Most of them are straight and are designed to be rotated in their long axis with a pronation/supination action of the hand to drive the needle through the tissues in a curved path. Mayo's is the simplest model, used in many modifications, similar in design to haemostatic forceps, with ratchet closure, and controlled in the same manner. Sir Harold Gillies (1882–1960), the New Zealand-born father of British plastic surgery, invented a non-locking combined needle-holder and scissors. Ophthalmic surgeons use a small holder for the fine stitching required.

1. Do not allow needles to come into contact with your skin but always hold them with a needle-holder, manoeuvring them within the needle-holder using dissecting forceps. Most needles are now curved but use the needle-holder to drive all types of needles through the tissues.
2. Grip the curved needle between the jaws of the needle-holder. The needle makes a right angle, with the holder. Have the needle point facing towards your non-dominant side and pointing upwards when your hand is in the mid-prone position, because you more easily drive the needle through by starting with your hand fully pronated, progressively supinating. This is a natural action whether you are inserting stitches from far to near or from dominant to non-dominant side.
3. If you are stitching in the depths of a wound, use a long-handled needle-holder, otherwise your hand is inside the entrance, blocking your view.
4. When you are inserting and tying stitches, or need to carry out some other short action, it is very convenient to palm the needle-holder. Remove your thumb from one ring, retaining your ring finger in the other. Swing the shaft of the needle-holder into the first interspace between the thumb and second metacarpal (Fig. 2.10) or swing it until it points back towards your elbow and flex your little finger into the space between the rings to retain it (Fig. 2.11). Do not retain the needle in the holder if you intend to palm it.
5. Occasionally you need to stitch alternately from right to left and then left to right, or far to near then near to far. To avoid the need to remove and replace the needle, merely turn it in the needle-holder, then turn the needle-holder through 180° in its long axis, and gain a fresh grip (Fig. 2.12).

RETRACTORS

These are extremely useful when you wish to display and carry out a procedure on a deeply placed organ. Some are hand-held, some are self-retaining (Fig. 2.13). For major abdominal operations a large metal ring may be placed

Fig. 2.10 Palm the needle-holder by removing your thumb from its ring, rotating the instrument on your ring finger, so that it lies in the interspace between the thumb and the second metacarpal. This slightly restricts movement of the thumb.

Fig. 2.11 Palm the needle-holder so that it points towards your elbow, and flex your little finger to lie between the rings, leaving your thumb and main fingers free.

to encircle the wound, to which can be attached various retractors. A retractor may be attached to a frame placed over the patient, to lift the lower sternum, improving access to the upper abdomen.

1. Use them carefully so you do not damage structures inadvertently. Ensure that the assistant who is retracting for you uses minimal traction and relaxes it whenever it is unnecessary.

Fig. 2.13 Retractors. **A** Hook. **B** Malleable copper. **C** Czerny. **D** Deaver. **E** Self-retaining. **F** Gosset self-retaining.

2. Exploit a change of approach: retraction by a hand placed over a pack is less damaging than a metal retractor. Sometimes a change of position of the patient or part allows gravity to produce the required effect.

CLAMPS

A wide variety of clamps fulfil the differing needs of grasping, joining and compressing structures (Fig. 2.14), and the mechanisms for fixing them vary from spring handles to ratchets, locking hinges and screws. As opposed to haemostatic forceps that are intended to clamp blood vessels that will be permanently sealed, bulldog clips and Potts artery clamps are designed to occlude them temporarily without damaging them.

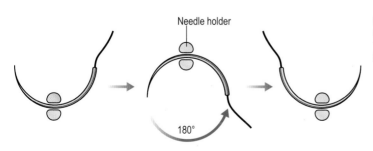

Needle holder

180°

Fig. 2.12 To reverse the direction of the needle, rotate it in the needle-holder, through 180°. This manoeuvre has been popularized by Mr W. E. G. Thomas of Sheffield.

Fig. 2.14 Clamps. From above there are four non-crushing clamps – bulldog, Potts arterial, intestinal, and Satinsky type; this allows part of the vessel to be isolated without totally obstructing the lumen. Below is a crushing, lever-action, intestinal clamp.

Fig. 2.15 Vascular clip. As you compress the clamp the clip first closes at the tips, preventing the enclosed structure from being squeezed out, before being compressed and occluded.

1. In order to prevent leakage of contaminating contents from the bowel, control oozing from the cut edges; to steady the ends while carrying out an anastomosis, many surgeons apply non-crushing clamps near the ends, including the vessels in the mesentery. In some models, the clamps on each side of the anastomosis can be fixed together. Other surgeons condemn the use of bowel clamps. Make up your own mind. If you do apply them across the mesentery, make sure you apply them very lightly, or just firmly enough to occlude the arteries. Do not merely occlude the veins while leaving the arteries patent. If you do so, the bowel and the occluded veins in the mesentery will become congested, may rupture and bleed into the mesentery, and be difficult to identify.

2. When you resect bowel you may place two crushing clamps side by side at each point of division and cut between them. In this way the cut ends are sealed. If you then intend to join the bowel ends do not fail to excise the crushed, sealed strip to expose the lumen.

HAEMOSTATIC CLIPS

Metal clips fit into the jaws of special forceps and can be applied across blood vessels and ducts to occlude them. The chevron shape ensures that as they close their tips meet first so that the tubular structure does not slip away (Fig. 2.15). Further compression occludes the lumen. Some instruments apply a series of clips from a mechanical or powered applicator. Another instrument applies two clips across a structure while cutting between them with a single action. Metallic clips are useful as radio-opaque markers to help identify their position after operation. They can be placed at intervals around a tumour in order to plan radiotherapy, and to estimate subsequent shrinkage as a result of treatment. Those made from titanium allow scatter-free computerized tomography and are magnetic resonance imaging compatible. A disadvantage of clips compared with ligatures and sutures is that they catch on hands, instruments and swabs and can be pulled off. Biodegradable clips are available as an alternative to metal clips. They are slowly absorbed.

STAPLING DEVICES

The principle of mechanical staplers in surgery is exactly the same as paper stapling machines. An inverted U-shaped staple is driven through the target tissues and then hits a shaped anvil that turns the ends (Fig. 2.16). The tissues should not be crushed because the ends are so turned as to form the shape of the letter 'B' lying on its face.

Straight staplers apply lines of staples, usually two offset parallel lines, and can be employed to seal, or seal and cut, tubular or vascular viscera (L = flesh or soft organs), and seal major blood vessels. A linear cutter applies four parallel lines and at the same time cuts along the centre to produce a double line of staples on each side of the cut. This can be used to produce a stoma between two segments of bowel. A miniature version of this instrument can be inserted through a laparoscopy port to doubly occlude a major structure such as a large blood vessel and divide it between the staple lines.

Fig. 2.16 The principles of stapling action. As you close the instrument you drive the staple points through the two layers of tissue before they impact on the anvil and are turned over to form the shape of a letter B lying on its face.

1. To unite two hollow viscera such as intestine, insert the limb containing the staple magazine into one bowel lumen through a stab wound and the anvil bar into the other bowel lumen through a stab wound.
2. Lock the two limbs together and actuate the instrument. When you unlock and remove the two limbs there remain only the two stab wounds to close, leaving a side-to-side anastomosis (Fig. 2.17).
3. Close the stab wounds with sutures or place a straight stapler across the everted edges of each of the holes and seal them.

Circular staplers (Fig. 2.18) produce an end-to-end anastomosis. There are two concentric offset rows of staples in the magazine head. At the end of a spindle is a removable circular anvil.

1. To form an anastomosis, insert the staple head through a side hole in the bowel wall, or, when performing a low colorectal anastomosis, for example, insert it through the anus. Fix the anvil on the end of the spindle, and introduce it into the other

Fig. 2.17 Linear stapler. **A** There are four lines of staples in the lower jaw, four matching lines of anvils in the upper jaw. Tissues can be placed between the two jaws which are then locked together. When the instrument is activated the staples are driven through the intervening tissues and folded over against the anvils. At the same time a knife is driven through the centre line of the staple lines, cutting the intervening tissues, separating them with each side sealed with a double line of staples. **B** A diagram shows how the staple lines are placed in the jaws with the anvil lines opposed to them. The knife will cut between the lines as shown in the end-on view.

Fig. 2.18 The head of a circular stapler. Two offset concentric rings of staples sit in the magazine with ends pointing upwards. The anvil has been unscrewed and turned towards you. When the anvil is reattached and screwed down onto the magazine, and the instrument activated, the staples are driven up through any intervening material or tissue and then bent over as they hit the anvil. A circular knife blade is also driven through, cutting off any protruding material or tissue, so the lumen is not obstructed.

end of bowel (Fig. 2.19). Insert a purse-string suture around each bowel end and tighten and tie them. This draws one end over the staple magazine end, the other over the anvil head.

2. Screw down the anvil to trap the two inverted bowel ends between the staple heads, without crushing them. Now activate the instrument. The staple ends are thrust through both layers of inverted bowel ends, hit the anvil and are turned over. Simultaneously an inner circular knife is pushed through to cut off the excess inverted bowel ends.

17

Fig. 2.19 End-to-end anastomosis of bowel. **A** Insert the staple head into the bowel through a side incision (or through the anus for a low colorectal anastomosis), pass it through the end and into the segment to be joined on. **B** Insert purse-string sutures round both ends and tie them to draw a ring of bowel end into the gap between the magazine and anvil. **C** Close the gap between the anvil and magazine to bring the peritoneal surfaces of the inverted bowel ends into contact. Now actuate the instrument to staple the bowel ends together and cut off the internal fringes of bowel. **D** After separating the anvil from the empty magazine, gently withdraw the stapler with a twisting motion before closing the side entry hole.

3. Now separate the anvil from staple head and gently withdraw the instrument with a twisting motion. Examine the trimmed ends encircling the central spindle. They should be complete toroids – 'doughnuts', confirming that the anastomosis has been perfectly carried out through the whole circumference. Check the circumference externally. If you created a side hole to insert the instrument, close it.

Skin staplers must be inserted without the presence of an anvil to turn the tips (Fig. 2.20). The central section of the U-shaped staple is held while the outer ends are pushed through the skin and then bent so that the ends meet, forming a closed ring. They are removed by straightening the base of the 'U' to open out the ends so that the staples can be withdrawn. Staples can be inserted from a magazine containing a number for convenience. The former clips devised by Gaston Michel of Nancy in France (1875–1937) have been virtually abandoned.

> **Key points**
>
> - Staples can be invaluable when stitches are difficult to place or are time-consuming in a major procedure.
> - Stitching remains the most versatile method of joining tissues.
> - As a trainee concentrate on acquiring suturing skill whenever it is convenient and safe to do so.

DISSECTION AIDS

You will, as a trainee, see a number of instruments used to aid dissection both in open and in minimal access procedures. Learn the principles of their properties and be aware of any side effects and dangers. They offer selective tissue destruction combined with haemostasis, and with varied penetrating effects on nearby tissues. There is a variety of instruments from different manufacturers, each with

Fig. 2.20 The principle of the skin stapler. Since there is no anvil beneath, against which to turn over the staple ends, the sequence is from left to right. The central column of the stapler has a lip beneath the staple to hold it. The outer parts thrust the staple ends through the skin and as they continue, the staple ends are forced to turn in towards each other.

its advantages and disadvantages – and new and updated products appear regularly.

> **Key points**
>
> - Do not attempt to use these complex and potentially dangerous instruments without proper understanding and training.

Electrosurgical dissection

Diatherm. The name should properly be applied to high-frequency electromagnetic waves as in a microwave machine. I have continued to use the term for the machine long used in surgery in which the electrodes are usually applied to the tissues, mainly to achieve haemostasis. For more recent, complex machines I have used the term electrosurgery. A high-frequency (400 kHz to 10 MHz) alternating current passing through the tissues between two electrodes may produce 1000°C heat.

Monopolar diathermy localizes the effect at the point of one (active) electrode, diffusing at the large indifferent plate placed in good contact, usually with the patient's thigh. The heating effect is greatest when using interrupted pulses of 50–100 per second, producing tissue coagulation into a semisolid mass, whereas a continuous current of sinus wave form vaporizes cell water, producing a cutting effect. A blend combines the effect allowing progressive dissection and haemostasis. For sealing bleeding over large surfaces an ionized argon gas flow can be used to complete the circuit between a monopolar diathermy electrode and the surface, spreading the effect.

Bipolar diathermy has the current passing only between the two tips of an instrument that encloses the tissues.

1. Diathermy is a valuable method of occluding blood vessels before dividing them, or sealing cut vessels. The combined action makes it a valuable dissector especially during minimal access procedures; a piece of tissue can be elevated with a hook, free of other structures, sealed and gently broken (see Ch. 13). By picking up the tissue with a bipolar forceps, the current passes only between the tines of the forceps, to produce a similar effect.
2. Beware the interference effects on pacemakers. Beware of using diathermy soon after applying spirit skin preparation, and in the presence of inflammable anaesthetic or bowel gas, for fear of causing an explosion. Do not leave the diathermy forceps or needle lying on the patient; keep it in its quiver when not in use.
3. Use bipolar diathermy whenever possible and stop diathermy if arrhythmia develops.
4. If the indifferent plate of monopolar diathermy does not have good skin contact, the skin may be burned. Test the connections and use short bursts whenever possible.

5. Capacitative coupling occurs if a metal object or instrument is near but insulated from the diathermy which induces a charge in the metal. Design changes have reduced the risk but beware also of bringing the electrode near another instrument.

> **Key points**
>
> - Do not apply diathermy for prolonged periods – the damaging heating effect spreads into previously normal tissues causing severe tissue destruction.
> - Do not apply diathermy to large tissue masses – take small pieces.
> - Prefer cutting, or combined cutting and coagulation.

Ligasure™ is able to seal vessels by compressing them between the jaws to obliterate the lumen, with computerized sensing of the collagen content, melting it and the elastin to create a seal. A knife can now be triggered to transect the tissue. It is claimed to be capable of sealing vessels up to 7 mm diameter with minimal charring and with very limited spread of heat into adjacent tissues.

Ultrasonic dissection

The mechanical energy transmitted by ultrasound can be used to disrupt tissues. If there is a high water content in the cells or tissues, it is vaporized, disrupting the parenchymal cells (G *enchyma* = infusion, inpouring: from ancient belief that the specialized cells were poured into the matrix scaffold and congealed), but sparing those with low water content such as blood vessels and ducts. At higher power levels, the vibration and resulting heat generation directly destroys cells.

Blood vessels and ducts can be sealed using ultrasonic energy provided the walls are flattened together within a clamp. The ultrasound energy produces heat to about 80°C; protein is denatured.

The *Cavitron Ultrasonic Surgical Aspirator (CUSA®)* consists of a titanium tube oscillating at 23 kHz which fragments tissue within 1–2 mm of the tip. The irrigation and suction facilities allow the fragments to be washed and sucked away. The parenchymal cells are disrupted leaving the vessels and ducts intact, so they can be sealed with ligatures, clips or other means, before being divided.

The *Harmonic Scalpel™*, producing 55.5 kHz, cuts using a hook dissector, or coagulates using a ball coagulator. Combined cutting and haemostatic vessel sealing can be achieved using low power. The vessel is compressed to appose the walls within a clamp, one blade of which is inactive, and the other is the ultrasound emitter (Fig. 2.21). Sealing is dependent on good vessel wall coaptation, low power and allowance of sufficient time for the weld to form. Claimed advantages over electrosurgical methods

19

Fig. 2.21 Principle of dissection combined with haemostasis by ultrasound energy. A vessel is compressed between the active and passive jaws of the clamp to appose the endothelial linings. The heating effect causes coagulation and 'welding' of the vessel walls, which seals it.

are that no electric current passes through the patient and heating of surrounding tissues is minimal.

Key points

- Dissection with electrosurgery or ultrasound both produce damaging heating effects, although less so with ultrasound.
- Dissection in layered tissue that can be separated into small bites causes minimal damage but dissection into solid organs and tissues presents the danger of creating inadvertent and macroscopically undetectable damage to important structures in advance of the dissection, which will subsequently undergo necrosis.

Miscellaneous methods

Laser dissection is widely used in various branches of surgery, employing variable wavelengths to suit the circumstances and the tissues involved. It is valuable for debulking large tumours.

Microwave dissection can be carried out using microwaves with a frequency of 2450 MHz to prevent bleeding.

Cryosurgery (G *kryos* = frost) is performed by freezing the tissues to −40°C with liquid nitrogen. Ice crystals form in the cells, disrupting them. The frozen tissue forms an ice ball which subsequently separates spontaneously from the surrounding tissues.

High-velocity water jet can be employed as a dissecting method since it selectively separates the tissues. Although it is not haemostatic, it disrupts loose parenchymal cells while leaving the blood vessels intact, which can then be dealt with by other means.

Radiofrequency tissue destruction is a valuable method of tissue destruction. An internally cooled needle delivers energy directly to the tissues to produce coagulative desiccation (L *siccus* = dry).

INTRAOPERATIVE DIAGNOSTIC ULTRASOUND

Mechanical waves above a frequency of 20 000 cycles/second (20 kHz) are inaudible to humans. Using low power intensity it can be valuable in intraoperative diagnosis, especially within solid tissues, such as liver, when deeply placed structures are impalpable. It can be used during open procedures and especially during laparoscopic operations since during these procedures the operator is precluded from palpating large organs or masses.

Chapter | 3 |

Handling threads

Threads of various materials are used extensively for ligating (binding) and suturing (sewing).

Manufacturers strive to produce threads that are strong, reliable, and produce minimal inflammatory, allergic or carcinogenic response. In some cases the threads are coated to improve the surface characteristics. Most threads are sterilized by gamma rays and presented in sealed packets.

All foreign materials inserted into the body evoke a reaction but some are relatively inert. Natural products tend to generate an inflammatory reaction, stimulating manufacturers to produce synthetic (G *syn* = together + *thesis* = a placing; hence, putting together) materials that are less reactive.

Threads may be absorbable and these are virtually all synthetic, predictably assimilated by hydrolysis, and so producing minimal inflammation. Non-absorbable threads are also nearly all synthetic including a polyamide such as nylon. The only commonly used natural thread is silk. 'Non-absorbables' almost always undergo changes within the tissues.

THREAD CHARACTERISTICS

1. Synthetic threads are usually extruded as a viscous substance through a fine hole, hardening to create a smooth-surfaced thread. A single monofilament thread has 'memory' which tends to make it return to its original straightness unless it is restrained, and since it has a smooth surface, loosely tightened knots tend to unfasten spontaneously. If the smooth surface is damaged by, for example, being roughly handled or grasped with a metal instrument, the thread is seriously weakened. Multifilament threads, made up of fine monofilaments, are virtually always braided, rather than twisted, so that when you roll them in your fingers they remain intact, instead of unlaying.

2. Absorbable threads may be monofilament or multifilament. Catgut is banned in many countries for fear of transmitting bovine spongiform encephalopathy (BSE). Synthetic absorbable threads evoke little reaction, and are absorbed predictably by hydrolysis, not by inflammation. Some slowly absorbed materials retain strength long enough to replace non-absorbable threads in certain circumstances. Monofilament substances include polydioxanone (PDS®), polyglyconate (Maxon®) and glycomer 631 (Biosyn®). Monofilaments, since they expose less surface to the body tissues, cause less reaction than do multifilaments and are preferable in the presence of infection because their smooth surfaces do not provide a nidus for microorganisms. Against this they are often difficult to handle and because they have smooth surfaces, knots do not hold so well. Multifilament threads, formerly often held together by twisting, are now almost invariably braided. They include polyglactin 910 (Vicryl®),

polyglycolic acid (Dexon®) and lactomer 9-1 (Polysorb®). These handle excellently, tie well, and retain their strength for prolonged periods. Do not pull them roughly through the tissues; their surfaces are not as smooth as monofilaments, so there is a dragging and sawing effect.

3. The only commonly used natural non-absorbable thread is braided silk, popular because of its soft pliability, and easily formed, reliable knotting. Polyesters, polypropylene and polyamides are synthetics and evoke minimal tissue reaction. Monofilament forms are strong but because of their smoothness, they do not bind together well and require multiple knotting to create reliable knots. Multifilament forms handle well and knot well. Stainless steel is favoured in some circumstances since it causes almost no tissue reaction – but it is difficult to handle. Have your assistant guide the loops of wire to avoid snags and twists.

4. Whatever the type of thread, do not use excessive force when pulling it. You may break it, but then, at least you are aware of this and can replace it. Worse, you may weaken it and it will break later. Do not drag it over sharp edges, or roughly snatch the strands together when tightening knots. Do not grasp threads with metal instruments except in sections that you will excise.

5. If you twist a slack thread it forms a loop (Fig. 3.1). Threads have an almost fiendish propensity to catch around the handles of surgical instruments or any other projection.

6. Surgeons vary in their choice of threads. As a trainee, note and use those chosen by your consultant. Make up your own mind so that at the completion of training you will have experienced a range of materials and can make a sensible choice.

7. Whenever you are handling threads arrange them so that they do not catch, remove all unnecessary

instruments from the area, or cover the projections with towels to protect them. If the thread becomes twisted when you are drawing it through the tissues, it may kink and cause damage, so run it through your fingers at intervals while the needle hangs freely, to allow the twists and possible snags to straighten out.

> ### Key points
>
> - If a thread frequently catches during certain manoeuvres, incorporate into your technique a routine to avoid it happening.
> - Do not wait for it to happen, to disturb your smooth progression, and then correct it.

Sizes

Thread diameter was formerly recorded as British Pharmacopoeia (BP) but is now usually quoted in metric gauge (Table 3.1).

KNOTS

As you read these accounts of knot-tying, have a length of string attached to a convenient base so you can practise the movements. This does not give you skill. It demonstrates what movements of the *thread* you must create. How you create them depends on your personal preference – what feels natural. You need to practise how best you can use your fingers, or instruments, to create them in differing circumstances and from different aspects. As you do so you create automatic movements that you can perform perfectly every time. Then, and only then, have you acquired a skill.

> ### Key points
>
> - Recognize that it is not sufficient to learn how to form knots. At least as important is how you tighten and bed them down while retaining the correct relationships between the threads within the knot.
> - In all these descriptions the loose ends are kept under complete control so that you do not need to look for them. They can be passed from finger to finger or finger to instrument.

1. A knot (strictly a bend or hitch, since a knot is a node or knob) is an intertwining of threads for the purpose of joining them. The ends of ligatures and sutures are joined in this manner. Secure fastening results from friction between threads and this is affected by the area of contact, the thread surface, the tightness of the knot and the length of thread left projecting from the knot.

Fig. 3.1 Effect of twisting a thread. Modern monofilament and braided threads do not unlay as did twisted threads.

Table 3.1 A comparison of thread sizes. The top line shows metric sizes, which if divided by 10, give minimum thread diameter in millimetres. The bottom line ('Others') shows the equivalent BP and BPC gauges, including both non-absorbables and synthetic absorbables.

Metric	0.1	0.2	0.3	0.4	0.5	0.7	1	1.5	2	3	3.5	4	5	6	7	8
Others	10/0	9/0	8/0	7/0	6/0	5/0	4/0	3/0	2/0	0	1	2	3&4	5	7	

2. The *half-hitch* (also called an overhand hitch) forms the basis of most knots used in surgery. Cross two threads to form a closed loop (Fig. 3.2). Pass one end through the loop. A half-hitch may be formed by crossing one thread over or under the other, thus making two forms of half-hitch possible (Fig. 3.3). The initial crossing may be left over right (on the left) or right over left (on the right).

3. If the two ends are to be tied in a half-hitch, they must be crossed and both tightened on the opposite sides of the knot from which they started (Fig. 3.4).

4. If you tie one half-hitch left over right and on top of it tie a second half-hitch also left over right, you produce a *granny knot* (Fig. 3.5). You could also tie two half-hitches right over left, right over left. A granny knot has much greater holding power than a single half-hitch.

Fig. 3.2 Forming a half-hitch. Cross the threads and pass one end under the crossing to emerge on the other side.

OR

Fig. 3.3 Two types of half-hitch: starting left over right or right over left.

A   B   B   A

Fig. 3.4 When forming a half-hitch the ends must be crossed and drawn in opposite directions. Note that end A starts on the left but ends on the right, and end B starts on the right and ends on the left.

Fig. 3.5 Granny knot. Follow the path of the threads; for the first half-hitch, the left thread was passed in front of the right one, then underneath, to emerge in front on the right side. For the second half-hitch, the new left thread (the former right thread) is also passed in front of the new right thread (the former left thread) and emerges in front on the right.

5. After tying one half-hitch, say left over right, crossing the threads so the left one is drawn to the right and the right one drawn to the left, create the second half-hitch by crossing what is now the right thread to the left over the left thread. This forms a *reef knot* (ON *rif* = fold; the knot used when folding and gathering a ship's sail to reef, or shorten it, in a strong wind Fig. 3.6). You could pass right over left, then left over right.

6. In the granny knot the threads of the two half-hitches cross rather than run parallel as in the reef knot, shortening the length of contact. Note the difference, by looking down on the knots. In a reef knot the ends lie parallel to the standing parts; in a granny knot the ends tend to lie at right angles to the standing part (Fig. 3.7).

7. If you create the same half-hitches as for a granny and a reef knot but keep one thread taut, you produce a slip knot. In the days of square-rigged ships, sailors

Fig. 3.6 Reef knot. The left thread was passed behind the right thread for the first half-hitch, then under it through the loop and taken to the right. The right thread emerges on the left. For the second hitch the new left thread passes in front of the new right and passes under it to emerge on the right.

Fig. 3.7 **A** Looking down at a reef knot. The ends lie parallel to the standing threads. In **B** the ends tend to project at right angles to the standing parts – this is a granny knot.

used the reef knot because it was not only secure but because it could be released easily and rapidly. Pull one thread straight and it produces a *slip knot* (Fig. 3.8). The two half-hitches can be slid off the straight, standing thread. This emphasizes the critical need when tightening the knots to maintain their relationship correctly.

8. After tying a reef knot, form a third half-hitch, creating a reef knot with the second half-hitch, to produce a *triple throw knot* (Fig. 3.9). This is even more reliable and is used as the standard method in surgery when security is essential.

9. The hands that control the ends must either cross each other, or exchange ends. If they are crossed in

the horizontal plane after the manner of crossing hands at the pianoforte (Fig. 3.10), they obscure the knot as they cross. If the hands pass each other in the sagittal plane, towards and away from the body (Fig. 3.11), the knot is not obscured at any time. You may be able to tie knots in the sagittal plane by adjusting your posture, either physically or mentally.

Fig. 3.10 Hands crossed in the horizontal plane obscure the field and are less in control.

Fig. 3.8 Two varieties of slip knot. **A** The result of pulling one thread of a reef knot straight – or keeping it straight while you form hitches round it. The other thread is converted to form two half-hitches round it. **B** The result of pulling one thread of a granny knot. Note that the other thread is converted to form the well-known clove hitch round it (clove = past participle of cleave, from OE *clifian* = to unite, adhere).

Fig. 3.9 Triple throw knot.

Fig. 3.11 Cross your hands in the sagittal plane.

Two-handed knot

I believe this is the safest knot. Why? Both hands are actively involved and sense exactly the tension on the threads, which must be even, ensuring that you do not distort the knot or pull on their attachment. At all stages you are fully in control of the thread ends, and of the direction and amount of tension, matching them on each side. It is a valuable facility to use either hand to form the crossing of the threads. If you are inserting sutures, holding the needle-holder in the dominant hand and using it to draw the thread through the tissues, you capture the short thread with the non-dominant hand. Right-handed surgeons hold the needle-holder with, and draw through the thread with the right hand. The left hand captures the short end.

1. If the short end of thread is towards you, capture it and hold it vertically between the thumb and index finger of the pronated left hand. Grip the longer end with the fully flexed right ring and little fingers, allowing the spare thread to hang from the curled little finger, leaving the thumb, index and middle fingers free. With your left ring finger draw a loop of the long thread to the left behind the short thread (Fig. 3.12).
2. Dorsiflex your right hand to thrust the pulp of the right thumb under the crossing of the threads, trapping the crossing between the thumb and the right index finger (Fig. 3.13). Release the grip of left index finger and thumb on the short thread to free it (Fig. 3.14).
3. Now palmar-flex your right hand, carrying the short end under the crossing of threads so that it points towards you (Fig. 3.15). Grasp the end once more between the

Fig. 3.13 Dorsiflex your right hand in order to place your extended thumb under the crossing of the threads.

Fig. 3.14 Trap the crossing with your index finger. Now release your grasp of the short end by left thumb and index finger. Prepare to palmar-flex your right hand, carrying the short end over and back under the crossing.

left thumb and index finger and take it away from you as you draw the long thread in your right hand toward you, to tighten the hitch (Fig. 3.16).
4. If the short end of the thread is away from you, pick it up between the thumb and index finger of the pronated left hand.
5. Grip the longer thread with the fully flexed ring and little fingers of the right hand, letting the spare thread hang from the curled little finger, leaving the right thumb, index and middle fingers free. Draw a loop of the long thread to the left in front of the short thread, using your left ring finger (Fig. 3.17).
6. Supinate and palmar-flex your right hand to thrust your index finger under the crossing of the threads, pointing towards yourself (Fig. 3.18). Pronate your left hand to draw the short thread pointing towards

Fig. 3.12 If the short end is near to you, hold it vertically by its tip, grasped between thumb and index finger of your pronated left hand. With the ring finger of your left hand draw a loop of the long thread to the left, behind the vertically held short thread.

Fig. 3.15 Your right index finger now pushes the short end under and towards you, as you release the loop held by your left ring finger.

Fig. 3.16 Grasp the end of the short thread between thumb and index finger of your left hand and carry it away, while drawing the long thread towards you with your right hand, to tighten the hitch.

Fig. 3.17 If the short thread is away from you, hold it up between the index finger and thumb of your left hand. Draw a loop of the long thread in front of the short thread with your left ring finger.

Fig. 3.18 Flex your right wrist and supinate the hand, to place the extended right index finger under the crossing of the threads and pronate the left hand to draw the end of the short thread pointing towards you.

you, and release it as you trap the crossing with your right thumb. Now fully pronate your right hand, carrying the short end under the loop to emerge on the other side, pointing away from you (Fig. 3.19).

7. Capture the end of the short thread again with your left index finger and thumb (Fig. 3.20) and draw it toward you as you take the long thread in your right hand away from you to tighten the hitch (Fig. 3.21).

8. If you start with the short end toward you, tie the hitch and carry straight on to tie the hitch with the short end pointing away from you. If you start with the short end pointing away from you, tie the hitch and carry straight on to tie the hitch with the short end pointing toward you.

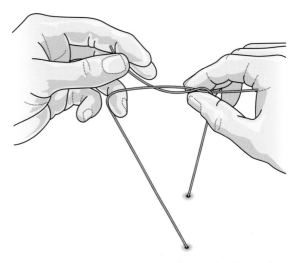

Fig. 3.20 As the short end emerges from under the crossing, pointing away from you, capture it once more with the left hand.

Key points

- How tight? This is most difficult to judge from watching experts, or for them to judge you.
- To ligate a blood vessel, just a little tighter than successful occlusion but not tight enough to risk damaging the integrity of the wall and risking separation of the stump. In an artery, not loose enough to risk pulsations rolling off the ligature.
- Tight enough to gradually cut through in the case of ligatures intended to cause ischaemic necrosis and separation.
- In living tissues, usually just enough to appose the tissues without blanching. Local oedema will later tighten the constriction and risk necrosis of the contained tissues with prejudiced healing.

Fig. 3.19 Trap the crossing of the threads with the thumb of your fully supinated right hand as you release the short end with your left hand. Fully pronate your right hand and extend the wrist as you carry the short end under the crossing, to point away from you.

Fig. 3.21 Draw the short thread toward you and take the long thread away to tighten the half-hitch.

One-handed knot tied with the left hand

This is a perfectly good knot, tied with the left hand, used effectively by surgeons while holding an instrument in the right hand. I deprecate its use by trainees who try to emulate the speed and elegance of experts without recognizing that although it is named 'one-handed' for forming, it is two-handed for tightening; in consequence they hold one hand still, form and tighten the hitches around it – and create a slip knot (see Fig. 3.8). Prefer slower, secure, two-handed knots unless you are confident that every hitch is

Key points

- If you are tying a ligature or suture in very delicate tissue avoid this knot. You cannot control exactly the tension you put on the standing parts as you hook your fingers round the vertically held threads to capture one of them.
- In contrast, you can form and tighten a two-handed knot while retaining exactly even tension, or no tension at all, on the strings as you form and tighten the knot.

not only formed but tightened perfectly every time, with crossing of the hands.

1. As with the two-handed knot, there are two types of half-hitch. When the short end is away from you, use the index finger (index-finger hitch). When the short end is close to you, use the middle finger (middle-finger hitch). The index-finger hitch and the middle-finger hitch must be tied alternately to produce a reef knot.

2. For the index finger hitch, when the short end is away from you, pick up the short end with the thumb and middle finger of the left hand and hold it vertically. Flex the wrist so your left hand hangs from it, then supinate your hand and extend the index finger to create a loop of the short thread over it.

3. Pick up the long thread with your right hand and hold it vertically in front of the short thread so that it crosses the short thread in the section between the index finger and the grasp of the middle finger and thumb of your left hand (Fig. 3.22).

4. Flex the terminal interphalangeal joint of your left index finger round the long thread to reach behind the short thread (Fig. 3.23). The short thread lies against your nail on the dorsum of the finger. As you pronate your left hand, extend the tip of the left index finger, carrying the loop of short thread under the loop of long thread (Fig. 3.24).

5. Release the middle finger contact with the thumb of the left hand to allow the end of the short thread to be carried through, and use the middle finger to trap the emerging end against the index finger (Fig. 3.25).

6. Now bring the short end toward you and take the long end away from you to tighten the hitch (Fig. 3.26).

7. For the middle-finger hitch, when the short end lies near you, pick it up between the index finger and thumb of the pronated left hand and hold it vertically. Pick up the long thread with your right hand and hold it vertically.

8. Supinate your left hand as you extend the middle finger between the near short thread and the far long thread and pull the long thread over it toward yourself (Fig. 3.27), crossing the short thread.

9. Flex the tip of your middle finger over the top of the horizontal section of the long thread and beneath the section of the short thread between the crossing of

Fig. 3.22 One-handed knot with the left hand. Hold the short end between the thumb and middle finger of the pronated left hand. Supinate the left hand, swinging the left index finger to push a loop of short thread behind and beyond the long thread held vertically in the right hand. This is the index-finger half-hitch.

Fig. 3.23 Flex your left index finger around the vertically held long thread so that you can pull a loop of long thread up with the pulp of the index finger, while the short thread crosses the nail.

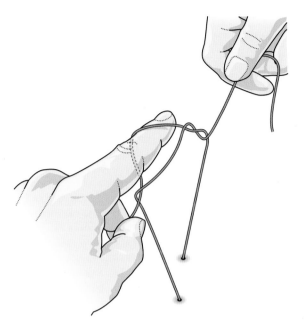

Fig. 3.24 While still holding the short end with the left thumb and middle finger, pronate your left hand, carrying the loop of short thread under the loop of long thread on the back of your index finger.

Fig. 3.26 Now draw the short end towards you and take the long end away to tighten the hitch.

Fig. 3.25 As the loop of short thread emerges, release the left thumb and middle finger grip on the end of the short thread and use your middle finger to trap the emerging end of short thread against the index finger to be replaced by your thumb.

Fig. 3.27 When the short end lies near to you, pick it up between the index finger and thumb of your left hand and pick up the long thread with your right hand. Supinate your left hand and extend your middle finger, behind the short thread. Draw the long thread over the extended finger from the far side, pointing toward you. This is the middle-finger half-hitch.

the threads and the grip of the left thumb and index finger; the nail of your middle finger lies in contact with the short thread (Fig. 3.28).

10. As you pronate your left hand, extend your middle finger (Fig. 3.29), to carry the end of the short thread underneath the long thread, to point away from you, as you release the grip of your index finger and

thumb on the tip, and extend your ring finger to trap the end against the middle finger (Fig. 3.30).

11. Now carry the short end away from you and bring the long end toward you (Fig. 3.31) to tighten the hitch.

Key point

- Note that when tying the index finger hitch you need to pick up the short thread between thumb and middle finger, leaving the index finger free; when tying the middle-finger hitch you need to pick up the short thread between thumb and index finger, leaving the middle finger free.

Fig. 3.29 Extend the terminal phalanx of your middle finger to carry a loop of the short thread away from you, under the long thread as you pronate your left hand.

Fig. 3.28 Flex the terminal phalanx of the middle finger, to pass over the long thread but behind the part of the short thread above the crossing of the threads. The nail lies in contact with the short thread.

Three-finger hitch. An alternative to the middle-finger hitch might be called the three-finger hitch.

1. When the short end lies near you, pick it up between the index finger and thumb of the pronated left hand and hold it vertically.
2. Supinate your left hand while extending the medial three fingers so that the short thread lies on the little, ring and middle fingers. Take the long thread over the middle finger from the far side and across the ring and little fingers, coming towards you (Fig. 3.32).
3. Flex the terminal phalanx of the left middle finger over the top of the long thread and under the section of short thread lying between the little finger and the grip of the thumb and index finger (Fig. 3.33). You can immediately trap the short thread onto the back of the middle finger, with the pulp of your ring finger.

Fig. 3.30 As the loop of the short thread emerges, release the end so that it is carried through; move your left ring finger to trap the end against the middle finger.

4. As you pronate your left hand, carry the loop of short thread under the long thread by extending the middle finger and ring fingers as in Fig. 3.29 and tighten it by taking the short thread away from you and the long thread towards you as in Fig. 3.31.
5. The advantage of using three fingers instead of the middle finger only, is that it is often easier to dip the terminal phalanx of the middle finger under the longer stretch of short thread. You can achieve this without exerting tension on the thread.

Fig. 3.31 Tighten the half-hitch by taking the short end away from you and drawing the long thread toward you.

Knot tied using instruments

Use instrument ties for repetitive routine knot-tying as when inserting a line of interrupted skin stitches. Do not use the method indiscriminately. When tying important knots revert to the two-handed method.

The method avoids the need to put down the needle-holder to tie two-handed knots. However, instruments can be 'palmed' – held by the medial fingers while using the lateral fingers to perform manoeuvres such as knot-tying (see Ch. 2) A less justifiable reason for using instrument ties is that the method is economical of suture material, since the short end need be only long enough to be grasped by the instrument, but this tempts you to hold it taut so the long thread forms a slip knot around it.

1. If the short end is away from you and the longer thread toward you, lay the needle-holder (it may be a haemostat or dissecting forceps – but I shall not continue to repeat this) on the long thread (Fig. 3.34).
2. Take the long thread closest to you and pass it over the tip of the needle-holder, round it, and back toward you (Fig. 3.35). While maintaining the loop, manoeuvre the needle-holder through it so you can grasp the short end (Fig. 3.36), and draw it back through the loop toward you, while taking the long thread away from you to tighten it (Fig. 3.37).

Fig. 3.32 'Three-finger hitch'. When the short thread is closer to you, pick it up with your index finger and thumb of the pronated left hand. Now supinate your left hand but instead of extending just your middle finger, extend the medial three fingers, allowing the short thread to stretch from the little finger to the index finger and thumb. Take the long thread in the right hand on the far side of the middle finger and lay it over the three medial fingers toward you.

3. If the short end is near to you, take the long thread away. Lay the needle-holder on top of the long thread (Fig. 3.38). Take a turn of the thread around it (Fig. 3.39), then grasp the short end through the loop (Fig. 3.40) and draw it through.
4. Tighten the hitch by taking the short thread away from you and drawing the long thread toward you (Fig. 3.41).

Knot-tying, using instruments only, has been brought to a fine art during minimal access surgical procedures but this is not a basic technique (see Ch. 13). Try practising the technique.

Laying and tightening knots

Key points

- Arranging the threads to lie in the correct relationship to each other is as important as forming the knots correctly.
- A carefully tightened knot weakens the thread significantly. A roughly tightened knot weakens it critically.

Fig. 3.35 Take a turn of thread round it.

Fig. 3.33 Flex the terminal phalanx of the middle finger over the long thread and under the short thread. Prepare to extend the middle finger to draw a loop of short thread under the long thread as in Fig. 3.29.

Fig. 3.36 Reach through the loop to grasp the short end.

2. This fault occurs particularly when you attempt to tie a knot when one end is short. To avoid losing it, you tend to keep it taut.

3. Once you have secured it, slacken it off until you have drawn the longer end through to match it. Plastic surgeons often pull the thread through when stitching, to leave a protruding end so short that when they have tied the knot they need to cut only the long thread. If you attempt to copy this technique take the greatest care to lay and tighten the knot correctly.

Fig. 3.34 If the short thread is farthest from you, lay the needle-holder on the long thread nearer to you.

1. Before you tighten a hitch ensure that the loops are of equal size. We automatically move our hands apart at equal speeds. If one loop is larger than the other, the shorter one tends to become tautly straight before the slack is taken up by the other (Fig. 3.42).

Fig. 3.37 Draw the short end through the loop towards you and take the long thread away from you to tighten the hitch.

Fig. 3.40 Grasp the short end through the loop.

Fig. 3.38 When the short thread is towards you, lay the needle-holder on the long thread lying away from you.

Fig. 3.41 Carry the short end through the loop and take it away from you while drawing the long thread toward you.

4. The force and direction of pull for both threads must be equal and lie along a straight line passing through the centre of the knot. Any other force or direction displaces the knot and puts traction on the attached tissues.

5. Carefully adjust the tension of the first half-hitch.

Fig. 3.39 Take a turn of the long thread around the needle-holder.

Fig. 3.42 When one end is short and you form a loop around it, then draw the short end through the loop, be careful not to tauten, and thus straighten, the short end. Allow it to remain slack while you take up the slack in the large loop through which it was drawn. On the left it is drawn out straight and a slip half-hitch results. On the right, the short end remains slack while you draw through the large loop to match it. Only then are the two ends evenly distracted to tighten a correct half-hitch.

Key points

- To appose tissues and encourage them to unite, do not over-tighten the stitch and constrict them.
- Remember that following a surgical procedure inflammatory oedema is inevitable; if the tissues are already constricted, they will die or the tie will cut out.

---

6. Conversely, when you are tying a vital ligature around a major blood vessel, if the tie is too slack it will be insecure. Tighten the second hitch fully onto the first. It is the binding effect of the threads of the two hitches that secures the knot.
7. When tying an important knot onto strong tissue, be willing to 'bed down' the hitches by gently and evenly tugging the ends apart two or three times (Fig. 3.43). Tighten the second hitch onto the first in a similar manner. Finally tie and securely tighten a third half-hitch, forming a reef knot with the second.

Tightening under tension

Of course we should not tie under tension – but we do not always have the choice.

1. If two structures must be brought together and held there with sutures or ligatures, use your assistant's hands to draw and hold them together while you tie the knots.

2. In order to create increased contact and therefore increased friction between the threads of the first half-hitch, pass the short end twice through the closed loop. When this is pulled taut, it has less tendency to slip than a normal half-hitch. Now tie a normal second half-hitch onto it to form a *surgeon's knot* (Fig. 3.44). I believe you should always tie a third, normal half-hitch, forming a reef knot with the second normal half-hitch.
3. A knot in which the second hitch also has two turns is sometimes recommended – and incorrectly called a surgeon's knot. When tying smooth-surfaced, extruded synthetic material, a number of methods are recommended, such as a surgeon's knot with a third hitch having two 'throws' or turns, or a standard reef knot finished with a third hitch also having two throws (Fig. 3.45).

Fig. 3.43 'Bed down' the hitch on a thick structure by gently pulling the threads apart several times.

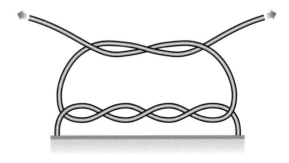

Fig. 3.44 This is a true surgeon's knot. The first half-hitch has two 'throws' or turns. The second is a standard half-hitch; I believe it should be finished off with a third half-hitch that forms a reef knot with the second half-hitch.

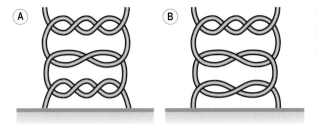

Fig. 3.45 Recommended knots for tying synthetic absorbable materials. **A** A double throw, then a single throw, followed by a double throw. **B** Tie a reef knot, then add a double throw.

4. If you are tying a thread around a structure that cannot be compressed by your assistant, such as a bulky elastic duct, then the thread itself must be capable of constricting and holding tight while you form and tighten a second hitch onto it. Try keeping the threads taut after tying and tightening the first half-hitch while you form the second hitch and tighten it onto the first (Fig. 3.46).

5. Particularly when suturing skin, the edges tend to separate after you have brought them together with the first half-hitch, which slackens while you are forming and tightening the second half-hitch. Try

rotating the threads clockwise or anticlockwise, to lock them (Fig. 3.47). They will lock only in one direction depending on which type of half-hitch you have tied. As you tighten the second hitch they unlock to form a secure reef knot but only if you form and tighten the second hitch correctly. Just as the second hitch tightens, it unlocks the trapped first hitch without giving it a chance to slacken.

6. If you deliberately keep one thread taut as you throw two half-hitches around it, to form a slip knot (Fig. 3.8), you can tighten it, to be held temporarily by the friction of the threads, while you now add two correctly formed and tightened hitches to make a reef knot.

7. An effective method of preventing slippage is to ask your assistant to compress the tightened first half-hitch with a finger while you form and tighten the second hitch, leading the tightening loop under the compressing finger (Fig. 3.48). Take care that you do not capture a small piece of the assistant's surgical glove, which will tear off when the finger is removed.

8. Another valuable method is to insert one or more temporary stitches to draw separated edges together while you insert and tie the definitive stitches, and then remove the temporary stitches (Fig. 3.49). You may tie them, or merely cross the ends and have your assistant hold them taut.

Tying knots in cavities

1. In some cases you need to tie a knot deep in a cavity. As a rule it is most convenient to form the hitches outside the cavity (Fig. 3.50).

2. Ensure that you have a sufficient length of thread so that after you have encircled or sutured the deep structure both ends of the thread lie outside the cavity.

Fig. 3.46 Tying a knot under tension. After tying and tightening the first half-hitch, keep the threads taut while you form and tighten the second hitch, to stop the first hitch from slipping.

Fig. 3.47 After tying and tightening the first half-hitch, rotate the ends clockwise or anticlockwise to 'lock' the threads while you tie and tighten the second hitch onto it. You must rotate the threads correctly and you must tie and tighten the second hitch correctly to create a reef knot.

Fig. 3.50 Tying a knot in a cavity. Form the hitches on the surface, so ensure the thread is sufficiently long.

Fig. 3.48 Your assistant's finger traps the first half-hitch while you tie the second half-hitch. You must lead the tightening threads under the assistant's finger – without capturing part of the glove.

Fig. 3.51 When tightening a knot within a cavity, you must push one end in with exactly the force with which you pull the other end out. If not, you will displace the structure, or pull off the ligature.

Fig. 3.49 Insert and tie a temporary stitch to take the tension while you insert and tie the definitive stitches. You need not tie it if you have your assistant cross the threads and hold them taut.

some cases when you can insert both hands you can pull the threads apart as you would on the surface.

6. If you merely pull on the deep structure you may damage it, or pull off the tie.

3. Tie a two-handed half-hitch outside the cavity (Fig. 3.51) without putting any tension on the threads.
4. With an extended finger, or a pushed but not grasping instrument, close the loop onto the structure.
5. Tighten the hitch by pushing down with a finger on one thread, with exactly the same force as you pull on the other thread from outside the cavity (Fig. 3.51). In

LIGATURES

A ligature (L *ligare* = to bind) is tied round a structure, most commonly a blood vessel or other duct, usually intended to close the lumen. Ligatures are secured by knotting the ends.

Key points

- Blood vessel ligation is one of the commonest repetitive procedures in surgery.
- Practise, practise, practise ligating vessels until you can perform it effortlessly, perfectly, every time.
- Perfection is more important than time. Indeed, two rapidly performed failed attempts take longer than a single effective ligature.

1. Silk is soft, flexible, can be tied securely without slipping and has a limited tendency to be reabsorbed. Avoid using it near the skin unless you will remove it, because it evokes a foreign body reaction, produces worrying subcutaneous nodules or even sinuses to the skin surface. It is sometimes attached as a marker to deep structures so they can be identified subsequently.
2. Synthetic polymerized absorbable threads are digested with minimum inflammation by hydrolysis. Springy stainless steel and synthetic non-absorbable material cause minimal tissue reaction but are usually now restricted to bonding together solid structures including bone.
3. Select the finest material that will reliably hold. Position it, tie and tighten it carefully. Too tight a ligature cuts through fragile tissue, too slack and it will not occlude a thick-walled vessel or it will slip off.
4. When preparing to divide and ligate ducts and blood vessels, preferably doubly clamp and divide them first or clamp them after they are cut. In either circumstance place the forceps with the concavity towards the cut and ensure that the tips of the forceps project a few millimetres beyond the ducts or vessels.
5. While an assistant holds up the handles of the haemostatic forceps, pass the end of the ligature under them on the side away from you, to capture it with the other hand (Fig. 3.52). Alternatively, stretch the thread between your hands on the far side of the forceps and then have your assistant reach over the thread and pick up the handles (Fig. 3.53).
6. When passing ligatures round vessels or ducts placed deeply, carry the thread stretched between the tips of your index fingers (Fig. 3.54) in order to reach under the tips of the forceps to avoid incorporating them in the ligature. Alternatively, use dissecting or artery forceps (Fig. 3.55) or an aneurysm needle. Warn your assistant to avoid pulling on the forceps; they will be pulled off or allow the ligature to slip over the tips of the forceps. Avoid tying in the tips of the forceps, or when they are removed, the ligature will be pulled off.
7. Tie the ligature carefully, slowly and securely.
8. Do not let your assistant undo all your safety precautions by cutting the threads too short. Have the ends of silk, linen, or braided materials cut 2–3 mm long, and monofilament materials cut to 4–5 mm.

Fig. 3.52 While your assistant lifts the handles of the forceps, pass the ligature from one hand to the other behind them.

Fig. 3.53 Stretch the thread between your hands beyond the forceps and have your assistant reach over the thread to pick up the handle of the forceps.

Fig. 3.54 Stretch the ligature thread between the tips of your index fingers to depress it and encircle only the vessel, without including the tips of the forceps.

Fig. 3.55 You may pass the ligature using long-handled dissecting forceps.

STITCHES

1. Versatile thread stitches are peerless for joining together tissues that can be pierced with a needle, in spite of the development of metal clips and adhesives. Threads are carried through by the needle and secured by knotting them.
2. Suture strength is related to the diameter of any particular material and is measured by the 'knot pull strength' test – the force that can be applied to the free ends of a suture tied with a surgical knot around a quarter-inch rubber tube.
3. A portion of tissue may need to be constricted to stop or prevent bleeding or leakage of internal fluids.
4. To prevent a ligature around a divided duct or vessel from slipping, first insert a stitch across the diameter of the tube, then tie it as a suture–ligature.

Fig. 3.56 Closing a defect. It was traditional, in order to avoid dragging the edges together under tension, as on the left, to bridge the defect with a darn as shown on the right. Because materials that are well tolerated by the tissues are now available, tension-free closure can now be achieved by inserting a polypropylene or similar plastic mesh extending beyond the margins of the defect, fixed with sutures or clips.

5. A stitch left long and untied can act as a means of exerting gentle traction. A coloured thread stitch makes a convenient marker.
6. If two materials are to be joined, insert the stitch through one, then the other, and knot the ends of the threads together.
7. A weak area or defect closed by inserting tightly drawn stitches has a high failure rate. Alternatively it was formerly reinforced by inserting a darn (Fig. 3.56), but polypropylene mesh, which is well tolerated by the tissues, has virtually replaced it. The mesh must be large enough to overlap the edges of the defect and is then sutured or clipped in place. A correctly inserted mesh creates a reliable tension-free closure of hernial and many other defects, replacing countless claimed methods that failed to live up to the claims.

Key point

- The more methods of dealing with a problem that exist, the less likely is it that any of them works reliably.

Needles

1. Needles come in a variety of shapes and sizes (Fig. 3.57). Curved needles are most commonly used. As a general rule they follow the circumference of a circle and may be but a small arc or more than half the circumference.
2. Straight, hand-held needles were formerly used extensively in surgery (Fig. 3.58). Surgeons are expert in handling them – flexible structures can be deformed in order to facilitate the entrance and exit of a straight needle to provide a curved passage of threads. The needles are so convenient that glove and skin punctures were accepted as a small price to pay. Recognition of the transmission of viral infections and possible prion diseases has made us change over exclusively to no-touch techniques.

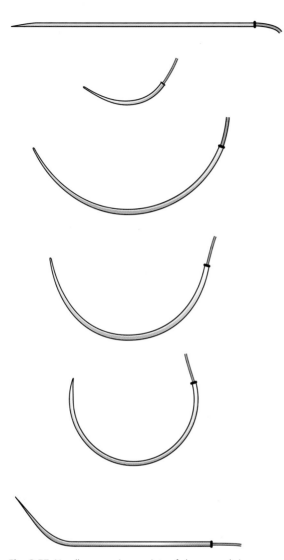

3. There are occasions when a straight needle is invaluable. Whenever you need to pass one always drive it by using a needle-holder (Fig. 3.59).
4. Virtually all needles are now eyeless and factory prepared. The needle is usually swaged onto the thread, although fine threads may be inserted and fixed with an adhesive into holes drilled into the shank of the needles. As a result the hole produced by the needle is only slightly larger than the thread that will be drawn through it.
5. Sutures are supplied in sealed packets after gamma ray sterilization.
6. A variety of points and cross-sections are available (Fig. 3.60) and the sizes range down to 3 mm for microsurgery. The needle shank is usually flattened along the section that will be grasped by the needle-holder.
7. Use a round-bodied needle to sew fragile tissue, or tissue arranged in strands that can be displaced since the strands are not cut, merely pushed aside, with minimal damage. Round-bodied needles are appropriate for sewing bowel and blood vessels because the round holes produced by the passage of the needle close by tissue elasticity around the thread, preventing leakage.

Fig. 3.57 Needles come in a variety of shapes and sizes.

Fig. 3.58 The hand-held straight needle is convenient – but dangerous.

Fig. 3.59 Insert and withdraw a straight needle using a needle-holder.

39

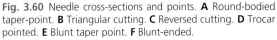

Fig. 3.60 Needle cross-sections and points. **A** Round-bodied taper-point. **B** Triangular cutting. **C** Reversed cutting. **D** Trocar pointed. **E** Blunt taper point. **F** Blunt-ended.

8. Skin and fibrous tissue are resistant, so use cutting needles of triangular or flat cross-section. The sharp edges of the needle cut through the tissues, so they do not contract onto the thread. Cutting needles of triangular section usually have the apex of the triangle on the inside of the curve. When such needles are used to insert stitches that will come under tension, in pulling two edges together, the threads tend to extend the split towards the edges with a liability to cut out. Reverse cutting needles have a flat surface on the inside of the curve and are less likely to cut out (Fig. 3.61). An alternative is a spear point, which is flat on the inside and outside of the curve.

Fig. 3.61 Closing a wound that is under tension or is liable to be put under tension. Top: the holes made by a standard cutting needle with the apex of the triangle on the inside of the curve. It is liable to extend when subjected to tension. Bottom: the holes made by a reversed cutting needle present a flat face to the site of possible tension when the suture is tied. There is less likelihood of such a suture cutting out if it is placed under tension.

9. Use blunt taper-pointed needles for stitching soft tissues such as the abdominal wall, excluding the skin. The needles penetrate the fascia and muscles but surgical gloves usually resist penetration and so protect you from needle-stick injury.
10. Use blunt-ended, round-bodied needles to sew soft viscera such as liver. Sharp-edged needles create splits that are likely to extend.
11. Use a robust trocar (F *trios* = three + *carre* = side) needle when sewing very tough tissues in which a normal needle might break.

Key points

- Do not pick up needles with your fingers. Use needle-holders and forceps to control them. Never leave them where they could damage your patient, yourself or your colleagues.
- When not in use, place needles with other sharp instruments in a kidney dish. Never pass them from hand to hand.
- Many needle pricks occur during abdominal wall closure; the blunt taper-point needle effectively penetrates the tissues of the abdominal wall but glove penetration is greatly reduced.

Stitching with a curved needle

1. Insert, drive and withdraw curved needles exclusively with instruments. The tissues can usually be moulded to conform to the curvature.

2. Do not select too short a needle. You need to have sufficient length to allow you to push in the needle and retain a grip until the point emerges sufficiently to be gripped without damaging the point. For the same reason do not attempt to take large bites of tissue on each side of a suture line in a single pass. Prefer to take the needle through each side separately.

3. Mount the needle in the tip of the needle-holder, approximately one-third of the way from the threaded end towards the point. If you are right-handed, with your hand in mid-pronation, the needle-holder pointing away from you, have the needle point upwards and to the left, upwards and to the right if you stitch with your left hand. Right-handed operators most easily stitch from right to left, and from away towards you. Left-handed operators prefer to stitch from left to right, and from away towards you.

4. Start with the hand fully pronated to enter the tissues perpendicularly (Fig. 3.62, see also Fig. 3.65A). As you continue, progressively supinate the hand so that the path follows the curve of the needle (Fig. 3.63). In this way the needle finally emerges perpendicularly from the tissues (Fig. 3.64).

Fig. 3.63 Needle driven in a curved path by progressively supinating your hand.

Fig. 3.62 Stitching with a curved needle. Start with your hand fully pronated.

Fig. 3.64 Your wrist is fully supinated as the needle emerges.

5. The ability to pronate and supinate enables you to drive a curved needle through the tissues with minimal trauma, and with minimal force. Make full use of this human facility. The range of movement can be extended by shoulder and trunk movements.

6. If necessary, use the closed tips of dissecting forceps to apply counter pressure near, but not on, the point of emergence of the needle in order to avoid turning the needle point and blunting it (Fig. 3.65A and B). If you use too short a needle, or take too great a bite, you may need to change the grasp of the needle-holder nearer the thread end of the needle, in order to push the needle further through. When the point comes

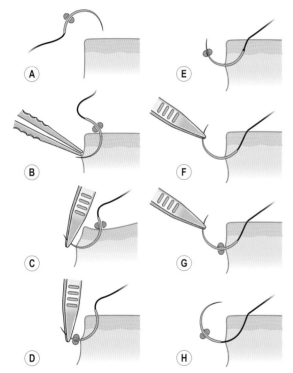

Fig. 3.65 Diagram illustrating the insertion of a stitch using a curved needle held in a needle-holder, indicated by two apposed stippled hemispheres. It shows a right-handed surgeon inserting the stitch from dominant to non-dominant side. If you are left-handed the needle is inserted in the opposite direction. **A** Enter the point at right angles to the surface; your hand is fully pronated. **B** As you drive the needle through, progressively supinating your hand, apply counter pressure against the tissues as the point emerges, so helping to reveal more of the needle. **C** When sufficient needle emerges, grasp and steady it with dissecting forceps. **D** Release the needle-holder and reapply it to the emerging needle. **E** Draw through the needle along its curved path. **F** Steady the needle with the dissecting forceps. **G** Reapply the needle-holder to the emerging needle at the place you wish to grasp it for the next stitch, keeping your hand partly supinated. **H** Finally, draw the needle right through, with a fully supinated hand.

into view, grasp the shank behind it, if necessary gently pushing back the surface tissue to expose a greater length of needle, and steady it (Fig. 3.65C).

7. Relinquish the grasp of the needle-holder and use it to re-grasp the emerging needle, gently pushing back the tissues to allow you to grasp it well away from the point (Fig. 3.65D).

8. Draw the needle through along its curved path (Fig. 3.65E) by further supinating your hand.

9. Again steady the needle with the dissecting forceps so you can disengage the needle-holder (Fig. 3.65F).

10. Re-grasp the needle in the correct position for making the next stitch (Fig. 3.65G), and draw it through (Fig. 3.65H). If you are inserting a continuous suture, this technique allows you to avoid the need to readjust your grasp of the needle with the needle-holder.

11. If you select the needle size correctly to match the tissue thickness and stitch depth and length, you can avoid several steps. In one movement you may expose enough emerging needle to be able to grasp it far enough back so that you can replace the needle-holder in the correct position for the next stitch. However, if you pronate your hand before grasping the emerging needle, you will need to change your grip before inserting the next stitch. Try it.

12. When stitching in difficult circumstances you may need to stitch from non-dominant to dominant hand direction, or from near to far. Sometimes you can avoid this by going to the other side of the operating table. If not, take especial care. You will be made aware of the difference in facility between making a familiar and unfamiliar manoeuvre.

13. Do not draw through the thread by pulling on the needle. You risk sticking the needle into an assistant or pulling the needle off the thread. Grasp the thread with a spare finger of the hand holding the needle-holder. Above all, do not draw through the thread by grasping it with the needle-holder or dissecting forceps; all the modern threads are severely weakened by being held with metal instruments.

14. Watch spare thread as you stitch. It has a fiendish propensity to catch on any projections. Have your assistant follow it and guide it; if you are using stainless steel you must avoid producing kinks. Do not try to stitch with thread of too short length – you are tempted to take shorter stitches, tie imperfect knots, and waste time.

Types of stitch (Fig. 3.66)

1. Surgeons often adamantly claim that the type of stitch they use is the reason for their success. They are too modest (a characteristic rarely attributed to surgeons). Their success depends on the care with which they insert the stitches, appose the tissues, adjust the tension and tighten the knots. Watch a few

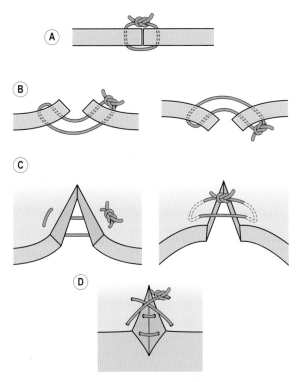

Fig. 3.66 Commonly used stitches. **A** Simple interrupted. **B** Interrupted longitudinal mattress, everting on the left, inverting on the right. **C** Interrupted horizontal mattress, everting on the left, inverting on the right. **D** Inverting 'X' stitch.

outstanding surgeons performing – the only common factor is the perfection of their technique, not the methods they use.

2. The simplest stitch to join two edges of tissue is a single thread that catches each side and draws them into contact, with both ends of the thread tied with a reef knot. This is an interrupted stitch. Pierce the tissue perpendicular to the upper and lower surfaces, otherwise it has an inverting or everting effect. If you tie it too tightly, or if it is subjected to too much tension, either the thread will break or it will cut out.

3. A mattress stitch is a double stitch. Start from one side, cross to the other side, reinsert the needle at a small distance from where it emerged and take it through to emerge on the original side a short distance from the first entry and tie the original entry and final exit thread together. If both stitches are parallel this is a horizontal mattress stitch. Because a mattress stitch draws on a segment of tissue between the two lengths of thread joining the edges, it is much less likely to cut out. This is particularly true when you sew tissues in which the fibres run at right angles to the edges. If the entry and exit holes are perpendicular to the edges, one bite is smaller than the other, this is a vertical or longitudinal mattress

stitch. In each case, there is a bridge of suture on the upper surface which draws in the surface away from the edge so that the edge itself is everted. These are therefore referred to as everting mattress stitches. Skin sometimes tends to invert and if you allow it to do so when closing a suture line, you are apposing the dead keratinized surface cells; healing is delayed and imperfect, so the scar will be weak. When suturing blood vessels you must appose the endothelium, by slightly everting the edges, or clots will form on the internal suture line. As a rule you can easily get the edges to turn out using simple sutures but on occasion you may need to start the necessary eversion with one or two everting stitches.

4. In contrast, bowel should not normally be everted. The French surgeon Antoine Lembert (1802–1851) recognized that if the outer, serous coats of bowel were brought into contact, they rapidly sealed together and prevented leakage. He described in 1826 a separate row of stitches that picked up only the serous and muscular coats, placed outside the main stitches, to create an inverting effect. However, the effect can be achieved with a single row of stitches and Lembert's stitch is less frequently used than formerly. Insert an inverting mattress stitch by passing the suture through the wall from outside in, to the mucosal surface, returning it to the surface on the same side a short distance from the entry stitch. Now cross to the opposite side and pass the suture from outside in to the mucosal surface, returning it to the exterior from the inside out, to emerge close to the entry stitch. Tie this thread to the end of thread at the original site. You have created a mattress stitch with the loop not on the surface of the bowel but on the mucosal aspect. When the stitch is tied it tends to bring the outer, serosal surfaces together. This stitch is often named after Gregory Connell, the American surgeon who described it in 1864.

Interrupted stitches

1. These have the advantage that when used in series, failure of one does not necessarily prejudice the other stitches.

2. The potential weakness of interrupted stitches is that each one is held by a knot; even when knots are perfectly tied and tightened they reduce the strength of the thread considerably. A roughly tied, snatched or imperfectly tightened knot may reduce the strength by over 50%. Once one knot gives way, the contiguous stitches are subjected to greater tension and may give way in turn. It is for this reason that you must form and tighten every knot perfectly, every time.

3. Moreover, tension on the stitches must be even, if they are not, the tightest stitch is exposed to excess tension and may give way, creating a domino effect. Furthermore, the over-tightened stitch tends to strangle the enclosed tissue and subsequently cut out.

Continuous stitches

1. These have the advantage of being quick to insert and have knots only at the beginning and the end – but those two knots are crucial.
2. Stitching can be carried out in a continuous manner, forming a spiral within the tissues. It has the advantage that the tissues are not strangulated, although the tension is usually sufficient to be haemostatic (Fig. 3.67A).
3. You may use a variety of stitches depending on the circumstances. If you pass the needle through the loop of the previous stitch before it is tightened, you produce a locked stitch, which holds the tension while the next stitch is inserted (Fig. 3.67B) – but do not drag the thread through the loop or you will damage it. A continuous mattress stitch with the

loops on the surface has an everting effect (Fig. 3.67C). In contrast a stitch leaving loops on the deep surface has an inverting effect (Fig. 3.67D).
4. In some circumstances it is an advantage to bury the stitches beneath the surface. This is especially valuable when you are sewing skin, in which case it is called a subcuticular stitch (Fig. 3.67E). I shall deal with this in more detail in Chapter 6.
5. When inserting stitches that will be buried in tough tissue potentially subject to tension, the required strength may demand a very thick, stiff suture that is not only difficult to knot but would produce a large mass of foreign material. By using doubled thread, the thickness can be reduced and the suppleness increased. Needles can be supplied with both ends of a thread swaged into the needle, leaving a loop at the free end. Make the initial stitch and pass the needle through the loop (Fig. 3.67F) so anchoring the thread with the minimum bulk. Continue the stitch and if there is sufficient length at the point of closure, cut one thread near the needle, take another stitch with the remaining thread and then tie the two threads to form a knot which is not excessively bulky.
6. When inserting continuous stitches, make sure they lie correctly; guide them by holding the loop with a finger or a closed dissecting forceps (Fig. 3.68) and carefully place the thread as you tighten it.
7. Continuous stitches cause twisting of the thread. From time to time run your finger and thumb along the thread from where it emerges from the last stitch to the needle to allow the twists to unwind, otherwise a kink may form and snag the thread.
8. The union may be edge to edge, inverted or everted, controlled by the way in which you form and tighten

Fig. 3.67 Continuous stitches. **A** Over-and-over, spiral. **B** Locking or blanket stitch. **C** Continuous everting mattress stitch. **D** Continuous inverting mattress stitch. **E** Subcuticular type of stitch. **F** Starting a continuous run using a doubled looped thread.

Fig. 3.68 Control the thread loop with your fingers or dissecting forceps as you tighten it, to guard against it snagging or catching on other structures and to ensure that it sits perfectly.

the threads and place the edges (Fig. 3.69). When sewing bowel, if you hold back each tightening loop while pushing in the edges with a fingertip or dissecting forceps, the loop will retain an inverting effect, especially if you tighten the thread only when you have inserted the stitch from without in and you are drawing the thread from within the lumen. This is because the tightening outer loop inverts the edges. When sewing skin or blood vessels, if you evert the edges between finger and thumb or dissecting forceps, the tightening stitch will retain an everting effect. Once started, the effect of edge-to-edge, inversion or eversion tends to continue as you insert further stitches.

9. At the beginning of the run, insert the first stitch and tie it as though this is an interrupted stitch, but do not cut the thread. Continue to the end. You now have two choices to tie off this single thread. The traditional method is to hold the last loop before inserting the final stitch, using the closed loop as though it is a single thread. Having inserted the last stitch, cut off the needle and tie a knot using the final thread and the closed loop; be careful and use several throws, since knots are not as secure using threads of different thickness as when they are the same thickness (Fig. 3.70). An alternative method is to hold the loop before the last stitch, then pull a loop of the thread following the last stitch through the first loop, tighten the first loop, pass a loop of the final thread

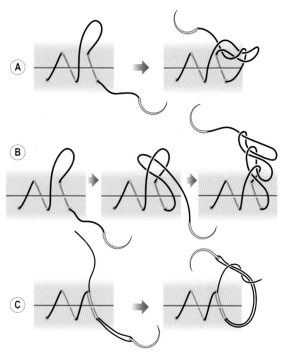

Fig. 3.70 Different methods of tying off continuous sutures. **A** Hold a loop before inserting the last stitch; use this loop like a single thread to tie to the end, after cutting off the needle – I have left it on in the drawing to identify it. **B** Hold a loop before inserting the final stitch. When you have inserted the stitch, pass a loop of the free thread through the first loop, tighten the first loop, pass a third loop through the second loop and tighten the second loop and so on three or four times. Finally, pass the needle and the free end through the last loop, tighten the loops and cut off the needle, leaving a generous free end. This is often called the Aberdeen, crochet, or daisy chain knot. **C** Very occasionally it is necessary to use an eyed needle. Hold on to the free end before inserting the last stitch, and tie this to the doubled end attached to the needle. Because the threads are of unequal thickness, tie several half-hitches and securely bed them down. Finally, cut off the needle.

Fig. 3.69 Producing inversion and eversion using simple 'over-and-over' stitches. **A** Push in the edges and hold back the loop with your index finger as you draw the loop tight from the under surface, along the line of stitching. **B** Alternatively, achieve the same effect by the 'no touch' method, using dissecting forceps. **C** Evert the skin edges using your finger and thumb. **D** Alternatively, achieve the same effect by gently pinching the edges to maintain the eversion.

through the second loop and finally pass the needled end through that loop and tighten it. This method is used by knitters finishing off a row of knitting as a chain stitch and by fisherman when they are repairing their nets – in honour of the fishermen of Aberdeen it is usually called an Aberdeen knot. Rarely, in order to insert stitches of an unusual material you may need to use an eyed needle. Hold on to the end of the thread before inserting the last stitch and tie this to the loop after making the stitch.

10. If you do not have sufficient thread to complete a continuous line of sutures, tie off and start again. You may leave the end of the first thread loose, insert a new stitch and tie it, then tie the loose end of the first thread to the new one.

Chapter | 4 |

Handling ducts and cavities

The body has a variety of ducts (L *ducere* = to lead or conduct). In addition there are many closed spaces or potential spaces. Be careful to avoid inadvertent injury to normal function:

1. Some ducts, such as the ureter, oesophagus and intestine, are capable of peristalsis. The circular smooth muscle contracts to occlude the lumen above, and relaxes below the content. An intramuscular neural plexus, named myenteric in the intestine, generates a wave of contraction preceded by relaxation, carrying the content with it. Consider the effects of any procedure on the resulting function. Other ducts, such as the common bile duct, have insufficient muscle to produce peristalsis and transmission of the content is by *vis a tergo* (L force from behind), often resulting from secretion into, and distension of, the elastic tube. In other circumstances transmission may result from external pressure changes; muscular expansion of the thorax expands the lungs and lowers the pressure in the trachea and bronchi, drawing air into the lungs.

2. Passage of content is often controlled by circular muscle sphincters, for example at the pylorus (G *pyle* = a gate + *ouros* = a watcher), at the anus and lower end of the bile duct – the sphincter of Oddi. There may be no anatomical, only functional evidence of a sphincteric action, for example at the gastro-oesophageal junction, which also selectively prevents reflux of gastric content into the oesophagus.
3. Although tubes within the body differ in form and function, they are all transmitters of substances which are absorbed from, secreted or excreted into, the lumen of glands, larger ducts such as the intestine, or to the exterior.
4. Passages and cavities are created by disease – sinuses and fistulas, or spaces such as seromas, haematomas, cysts and abscesses. Potential spaces are opened up surgically. Artificial fistulas include internal fistulas such as gastroenterostomy and external stomas (G *stoma* = a mouth).
5. Wherever there is stagnation in spaces or in ducts, microorganisms collect and tend to contaminate and infect the tissues.
6. Ducts and cavities are prone to injury, stenosis, obstruction, other mechanical problems, or paralysis, and require intubation, dilatation, drainage, repair and anastomosis. Some cavities require similar management.
7. The principles of management are often common to different situations. For this reason, acquire familiarity with all the techniques, watch experts, and assiduously practise the manoeuvres to develop the necessary skills. Success often results from adapting methods from one area to another.
8. I have used as examples, procedures that are life-saving or commonly performed, to demonstrate the required technical skills – but have excluded selection, preparation and aftercare.

INTUBATION

Percutaneous intubation

A number of commonly performed procedures, some of them life-saving, incorporate percutaneous (L *per-* = through, beyond + *cutis* = skin) puncture.

1. Insert needles in a straight line; if you need to change direction it is usually better to withdraw the needle and reinsert it. If you move the needle within the tissues you risk damaging any or all of the structures between the entry point and the tip.
2. Hollow needles are available in varying diameters and lengths; for example, long thin 'skinny' needles are used for percutaneous liver puncture to minimize subsequent leakage. Needles are usually best connected to a syringe so that you can see what emerges, or aspirate contents. Do not use short needles that must be fully inserted, since if they break off at the Luer connection, the thin retained shaft is difficult to identify and grasp.
3. When you intend to remove fluid, it may be convenient to interpose a three-way tap between the needle and the syringe; aspirated fluid can then be expelled through the side channel of the tap, into a receiver.
4. Some needles have an internal obturator (L *obturare* = to stop up) that is withdrawn when the needle is correctly placed, allowing contents to emerge; lumbar puncture needles have stylettes, presumably to prevent the contamination of cerebrospinal fluid by other fluids during the passage of the needle.
5. If you wish to inject fluid into a tube or space, can you confirm that the tip of the needle is correctly sited? You may aspirate identifiable fluid into a syringe attached to the needle. To minimize subsequent leakage along the needle track when performing percutaneous transhepatic biliary puncture, a long, very thin, 'skinny' needle is used. Bile can be aspirated and radio-opaque material injected to outline the biliary tract radiographically (Fig. 4.1A). You may aspirate fluid from a cyst, blood from a haematoma or pus from an abscess cavity (Fig. 4.1B). In some cases, ease of fluid injection helps confirm that the tip is in the correct place; for example, insufflation (L *in* + *sufflare* = to blow) of

Fig. 4.1 A Percutaneous puncture to gain access to ducts. To guard against subsequent leakage from, for example bile ducts within the liver, a long, thin 'skinny' needle is used. **B** Puncture of a cavity such as a cyst, haematoma or abscess cavity.

the peritoneal cavity with carbon dioxide to initiate pneumoperitoneum does not produce a rapid rise in pressure as would occur if the gas is infused into a closed space. In contrast, when you wish to inject into a closed space such as an obstructed tube, carefully note if the flow is freer than you expect, suggesting you have entered an extensive cavity.

6. When you have entered the tube or space, make sure you do not penetrate beyond it. One method is to mark the penetrator with a clamp or the sterile-gloved fingers, or use a penetrator with a shoulder such as on a haemorrhoid injection needle, to limit its entrance. A similar risk occurs when creating a pneumoperitoneum prior to minimal access surgery (see Ch. 13). To minimize the risk of penetrating the viscera within the potential space before they fall away from the parietal peritoneum (see Fig. 4.2 and Ch. 13), use the special Veress needle which has a sharp bevel tip but within it is a spring-loaded blunt trocar. As soon as the bevel penetrates the parietal peritoneum the trocar projects, pushing away any at-risk viscera. In other circumstances you may not know the required depth of penetration; when entering the trachea, too deep intrusion may damage the thin posterior wall or even breach the oesophagus. Too deep insertion of the needle may cause damage during lumbar puncture or pericardiocentesis.

Cricothyroid puncture may be life-saving in the absence of any other means of relieving respiratory obstruction.

1. Feel for the laryngeal prominence, follow down the anterior edge of the thyroid cartilage to the gap between the thyroid and cricoid cartilages, identifying the cricothyroid membrane (Fig. 4.3).

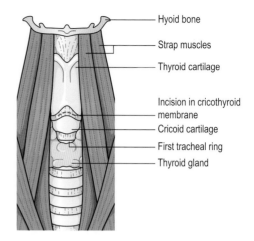

Fig. 4.3 Cricothyrotomy. The incision is shown in the broken line.

2. Insert a needle carrying an external cannula, in the midline just above the cricoid cartilage, aiming slightly caudally, while aspirating on an attached syringe. Feel for the 'give' as you pierce the cricothyroid membrane. As soon as air enters the syringe you are in the trachea.
3. Hold the needle still, while gently advancing the cannula. If you do not have a cannulated needle, insert one or more plain needles to create an emergency short-term relief.

Cricothyrotomy is the preferred emergency procedure.

1. Carry it out if necessary without preliminary local anaesthesia and tracheal intubation.

Fig. 4.2 Methods of limiting overpenetration and inadvertent damage to susceptible structures. **A** Place a non-damaging clip on the puncturing instrument. **B** Use a shouldered needle, as is used for injection of haemorrhoids. **C** Grasp the instrument at a point that limits insertion. **D** The Veress needle has a blunt, spring-loaded obturator that projects as soon as resistance is overcome, pushing away at-risk mobile structures.

2. Place the patient supine, head straight, in line with the body. If possible extend the neck by placing a pillow under the upper thoracic spine.
3. Ensure that the trachea is central. Identify the thyroid cartilage. Follow the anterior border down to the gap from here to the cricoid cartilage.
4. Incise the skin transversely for 1–1.5 cm over the centre of the cricothyroid membrane and deepen it down to and through the membrane, signalled by a hiss of air.

Key points

- Do not extend the incision too far laterally or you may cause bleeding from the anterior jugular veins.
- Avoid inserting the knife too deeply or you may penetrate the thin posterior wall into the pharynx.

5. It was traditional to reverse the knife, insert the handle into the laryngeal incision and turn it to open the incision, but in doing so you may not succeed in relocating and re-entering the larynx. Hold the knife blade quite still and insert alongside it a haemostatic or other forceps. Now withdraw the knife blade, open the forceps to create a gap and insert the tracheostomy tube alongside it. If you do not have a tracheostomy tube use whatever is available. Remove the forceps. If the tube has an inflatable cuff, gently expand it. If it has attached tapes, encircle the neck and tie them to secure the tube. Use your ingenuity to fix an improvised tube.

Key points

- In an emergency use your ingenuity. Many lives have been saved using penknives to insert a variety of tubes.
- Tracheostomy is inappropriate as an emergency procedure except by an expert.

Lumbar puncture is usually performed with the patient lying on the side, strictly horizontal, parallel to the couch, with fully flexed spine to widen the space between the posterior vertebral arches. Have a receptacle available to collect cerebrospinal fluid if this is a diagnostic procedure.

1. Under strict sterile precautions, following an injection of local anaesthetic, insert the spinal needle with the lumen filled by stylette, between the third and fourth, or fourth and fifth lumbar vertebral spines, perpendicular to the skin surface or minimally angled in a cephalic direction. A line joining the highest points of the iliac crests on each side passes through the spines of the fourth and fifth vertebrae.

2. Feel for the 'give' as you pierce the interlaminar ligament (ligamentum flavum) – the depth for extradural – 'epidural' – puncture.
3. If you need to enter the subarachnoid space, carefully feel for the second, less obvious 'give' as you pierce the dura – the arachnoid mater is closely applied to the undersurface of the dura of the spinal canal.
4. Withdraw the stylette to watch for cerebrospinal fluid to emerge from the needle, and collect a specimen for biochemistry and bacteriology.

Pericardiocentesis (G *kentesis* = puncture) should be performed with electrocardiographic monitoring.

1. Insert the needle, connected through a three-way tap to a capacious syringe, just to the left of the xiphisternum, aimed towards the tip of the left scapula. Be sensitive to the 'give' as you puncture the pericardium, then aspirate to draw fluid into the syringe.
2. If you irritate the myocardium by contact with the needle you will provoke cardiac irregularities.

Suprapubic cystostomy is an example of the value of distending a tube or cavity in order to enter it. A traditional method is to use a trocar (F *trios* = three + *carre* = side, since the sharp tip of the internal perforator was three-sided), and cannula (Fig. 4.4).

1. Carry it out with strict sterile precautions.
2. Ensure that the bladder is full, confirmed by displaying suprapubic dullness to percussion. Bladder distension peels the peritoneal reflection from bladder wall to abdominal wall upwards, and so avoids the risk of puncturing the peritoneal cavity (Fig. 4.5).

Ⓐ Ⓑ

Fig. 4.4 A A traditional trocar, a cannula, and then the trocar fitted into the cannula. **B** A cross-section of a disposable Lawrence-type trocar and cannula, together with a close-up view of the thin panel being stripped along the length of the cannula so that it can be detached from the catheter that has been inserted through it.

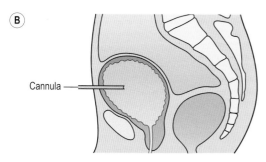

Fig. 4.5 Suprapubic cystostomy. In **A** the bladder is empty. A cannula inserted into the bladder is at risk of transgressing the peritoneal cavity. In **B** the bladder is full and the peritoneal reflexion from the anterior abdomen onto the bladder is well above the track of the cannula.

3. Infiltrate the skin with local anaesthetic in the midline, 3–5 cm above the symphysis pubis. Using a longer needle, inject down to and into the bladder wall. When there is a sudden 'give' and you can aspirate urine, you have entered the bladder. Do not continue unless you have confirmed this.

4. Withdraw the syringe and needle. Make a short incision with a scalpel at the site of needle entry and carefully cut vertically down to the bladder wall.

5. Gently insert the trocar and cannula along the prepared track and through the bladder wall into the lumen. Avoid sudden uncontrolled penetration that might endanger pelvic structures.

6. Withdraw the trocar, at which point urine should emerge. Immediately insert a Foley catheter through the cannula.

7. When you are confident that the tip and balloon are in the bladder, carefully remove the cannula without displacing the catheter and inflate the catheter-retaining balloon. A traditional cannula may resist being withdrawn over the bulky catheter outlet. The disposable plastic Lawrence-type cannula has a detachable strip so that it can be opened out to detach it after withdrawing it from the bladder (Fig. 4.4).

8. Attach the catheter to a drainage tube emptying into a collecting bag. The wound requires only a simple, temporary dressing.

Peritoneal diagnostic lavage is useful if ultrasound or computerized tomography imaging are unavailable to determine whether or not there is intra-abdominal damage. It is an alternative to diagnostic laparoscopy.

1. Pass a urinary catheter and nasogastric tube to ensure that the bladder and stomach are empty. Have a specimen tube and culture swab available in case any fluid emerges.

2. Under sterile conditions, after infiltrating local anaesthetic, make a 2 cm vertical incision at the junction of the upper third and lower two-thirds of the line joining the umbilicus and symphysis pubis, down through the linea alba to the peritoneum. Carefully pick up and lift the peritoneum between two pairs of forceps and incise it to gain access to the peritoneal cavity.

3. Insert a finger to ensure that you have safely entered the abdomen and pass in the end of a dialysis catheter, guiding it down towards the pelvis. Connect a syringe and aspirate the catheter, sending any aspirate for microscopy.

4. Connect the tube to a container of Ringer/lactate solution, 10 mL/kg body weight, warmed to body temperature, and slowly run it into the abdomen (Sydney Ringer, 1835–1910, was an English physiologist).

5. Gently agitate the abdomen, wait for 10 minutes, then lower the container to the floor, allowing the fluid to siphon back into the bag. Send a specimen for microscopy.

6. The test is positive if there are more than 100 000 red cells and more than 500 white blood cells per cubic millimetre, making it likely that there is intra-abdominal damage.

Chest drain allows you to remove air or liquid to achieve and maintain lung expansion (see Ch. 11).

> **Key points**
>
> - Do not wait to insert a chest drain in the presence of tension pneumothorax.
> - Introduce needles, or make an intercostal incision just above a rib into the pleural cavity, converting it to a simple pneumothorax, releasing the tension.

Direct intubation

1. Ducts, tubes, and spaces that open onto the surface, or are exposed at operation, can be intubated directly.

2. By special techniques internal ducts may be cannulated through instruments such as endoscopes, which are usually passed into hollow viscera via

natural orifices. For example, the common bile duct or pancreatic duct can be cannulated through a fibreoptic upper gastrointestinal endoscope, the ureter can be catheterized through a cystoscope. I shall not describe these since they require special training.

3. Plastic, latex rubber, metal, and in the past gum elastic and other types of catheters have been used, having plain open ends, side holes, and with straight or curved tips (Fig. 4.6). Choose one that slips in easily without being gripped by the walls or you will lose the 'feel' of the catheter. Ducts that can be directly intubated include the trachea, urethra, upper and lower gastrointestinal tracts, salivary ducts, stomas, external sinuses and fistulas, or ducts exposed at operation.

Fig. 4.7 Twist the catheter back and forth between thumb and forefinger to allow it to search out the channel.

Key points

- If you have difficulty in advancing a tube or catheter through a convoluted space, do not use force.
- Slightly withdraw it and rotate it before gently advancing it again (Fig. 4.7).
- In case of difficulty, twist a flexible catheter back and forth between finger and thumb to allow it to search out the channel.
- When possible apply gentle traction to straighten the channel.

---

1. Choose an endotracheal tube of the correct length and diameter and test the inflatable cuff. Lubricate the tube with water-soluble jelly.
2. Place the patient supine with a small cushion under the shoulders. Keep the neck straight in the line of the body, slightly flexed, with the head extended at the atlanto-occipital joint, resting on a small pillow.
3. The path the tube will take is a curved one, but you must control it under direct vision; this entails temporarily straightening it. Achieve this by using a Mackintosh laryngoscope (Fig. 4.8), held in the non-dominant hand.
4. The mouth and opening of the larynx lie anteriorly but the base of the tongue and epiglottis bulge posteriorly. Lift them, and the mandible, by placing the 'beak' of the laryngoscope in the vallecula (L diminutive of *vallis* = valley) between the tongue base and the epiglottis, and gently raise them.

Tracheal intubation can be carried out through the mouth or through the nose, although nasal intubation requires special skill. You will normally pass an endotracheal tube only on a deeply unconscious patient.

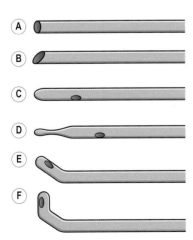

Fig. 4.6 Catheter tips. **A** Open end. **B** Flute tip. **C** Round end with side hole. **D** Olivary tip. **E** and **F** Coudé and bicoudé (F = bent and double-bent).

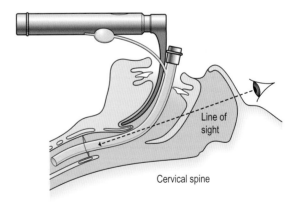

Fig. 4.8 Insertion of an endotracheal tube. The base of the tongue and epiglottis are raised with Mackintosh's laryngoscope. You would be looking past one side of the nose and through the side of the mouth to see the laryngeal opening. The curved endotracheal tube can now be inserted under vision.

5. You can now look from the head of the table along one or other side of the nose and view the pharynx and laryngeal opening through the side of the mouth, alongside the tongue (Fig. 4.8).
6. Pass the tube of correct diameter, length and curvature, under vision, through the laryngeal opening into the trachea. The inflatable cuff must lie beyond the vocal cords; gently expand it through the side tube just enough to completely fill the trachea.
7. Check the pressure in the cuff by feeling the small monitor balloon on the inflation tube, then clamp the tube. Collapse of this balloon warns you if the cuff leaks and deflates.
8. Now check that if the chest is compressed air is ejected through the endotracheal tube; if the tube is connected to a bag which is then compressed, the chest should expand – but ensure that the tube does not lie in the oesophagus by excluding upper abdominal distension or an epigastric tympanitic note on percussion.

Feeding jejunostomy is an example of a catheter introduced through the abdominal wall, then into the intestine, when the abdomen is open.

1. Place a large haemostat or tissue forceps with which to lift the left wound edge. Make a stab incision through the abdominal wall in the left upper quadrant of the abdomen well clear of the abdominal incision, umbilicus and the rib margin. Take great care to avoid injuring the intra-abdominal structures.
2. Evert the wound edge and pass a haemostat through the stab wound from within out, to grasp the tip of the catheter and draw it into the abdomen.
3. Lift the greater omentum and left transverse colon. Identify a suitable segment of proximal jejunum by finding the ligament of Treitz and following the bowel distally until you have a loop long enough to reach the anterior abdominal wall without tension.
4. On the antimesenteric border, encircle the intended catheter entry site with a seromuscular purse-string suture tied but slack. Make a small incision within the relaxed purse-string, taking care to avoid cutting the suture. Insert the tip of the catheter through the hole, pointing distally for 10 cm. Tighten and tie the purse-string but not sufficient to obstruct the catheter. You may insert a further purse-string suture, inverting the first one to create an ink-well effect.
5. Leave the purse-string suture ends long and take them back and forth around the emerging catheter (see below), tying them to hold the catheter in place.
6. Evert the abdominal wall to facilitate inserting three to four stitches, each one catching the seromuscular coat of the jejunum close to the emerging catheter and the parietal peritoneum near the stab wound in the abdominal wall. Place all the stitches, then gently tighten them to draw the jejunum into contact with the abdominal wall, forming a seal.

7. After closing the abdominal wall, place a stitch through the skin near the emerging catheter, tie it, then encircle the catheter and tie it again so that any traction on the catheter does not displace it, but is taken by the stitch.
8. Now close the abdomen.

Urethral catheterization in the male is a classical example of the art of inserting tubes, because it demands great sensitivity, gentleness and skill.

1. Carry out the procedure under strict sterile precautions. Check that you have available an appropriate catheter, usually Foley self-retaining (e.g. 16–18 F) with the inner sterile plastic container opened but the catheter unexposed, a local anaesthetic tube of 2% lidocaine (lignocaine) hydrochloride gel and sterile nozzle, forceps, towels, swabs, mild aqueous antiseptic solution, water-soluble lubricant, urine receptacle, tubing and collecting bag. Have a syringe and sterile fluid available if you are inserting a Foley-type catheter.
2. Place the patient supine, thighs separated, pudenda exposed. With a sterile swab held in your non-dominant hand grasp the loose dorsal skin of the penis just behind the corona. With another swab held in your dominant hand, clean the head and corona, pushing back the uncircumcised foreskin to expose the glans.
3. Hold up the penis and apply sterile towels – usually a single disposable sheet with a hole in the middle. Replace your grasp with a fresh swab folded lengthwise as a sling that can be held, together with a fold of loose dorsal skin, just behind the corona, between finger and thumb of the non-dominant hand (Fig. 4.9), leaving the other fingers free. Again swab the meatus and penile head with antiseptic solution.
4. Insert the anaesthetic through the nozzle and occlude the urethra to retain it for at least 3–4 minutes by compressing the undersurface of the penis through the sling-like swab, using the medial fingers of your non-dominant hand.
5. Draw the penis vertically upwards, thus straightening the penile urethra (Fig. 4.10). Manipulate the opened inner sterile plastic catheter container to allow 5–7 cm of the tip to protrude. Do not touch the catheter but hold and control it through the cover. Lubricate and insert the catheter tip gently and slowly. Progressively draw back the plastic container.
6. Prevent the catheter from being extruded following each advancement by wrapping the free fingers of the left hand around the ventral surface covered by the enfolding sterile swab and compressing the urethra against the catheter. The catheter sometimes passes through the sphincter into the bladder if you are patient.
7. If the catheter is held up, draw the penis towards the feet. Without losing your grip on it, swing the penis down between the separated thighs. This has the

Fig. 4.9 Grasp the penis in a gauze swab sling placed just proximal to the corona. Grip the swab and a fold of loose dorsal skin between finger and thumb, leaving the other fingers free to wrap around the penis to compress the urethra during catheterization to prevent the catheter from being extruded.

effect of directing the tip of the catheter upwards into the prostatic urethra and bladder.

8. Ensure that the catheter can empty into a container. Now gently advance it through the prostatic urethra into the bladder. Success is signalled by the appearance of urine. If no urine emerges when the catheter seems to be fully inserted, try pressing on the bladder suprapubically through the sterile towel. Maintain compression of the urethra to prevent the catheter from being extruded until you have secured it by inflating the balloon.

9. Obtain a specimen of urine for microscopy and culture, then connect the catheter to a closed collecting bag.

Fixing catheters and tubes

Various tubes fulfil an important and sometimes life-saving function. Make sure that you fix them securely and safely. Replacing a catheter that has been inserted with great difficulty and has now fallen out is challenging – both for you and for the patient.

Self-retaining catheters. In the past rubber catheters were moulded with projections that could be straightened by stretching or compressing during insertion but they have been largely superseded by the invention of the American urologist Frederic Foley of Minnesota (1891–1966), which is an inflatable balloon near the tip of the catheter (Fig. 4.11); the catheter can be withdrawn easily after deflating the balloon. A useful retaining device within a small duct is the 'T'-tube catheter (Fig. 4.12). The short limb of the 'T' lies

Fig. 4.10 A Hold the shaft of the penis dorsally, just behind the corona. First pull it vertically to straighten the penile urethra while you insert the catheter as far as the bulb. **B** Now draw the penis down towards the feet to align the penile and membranous parts of the urethra.

Fig. 4.11 Self-retaining catheters. **A** Foley catheter with an inflatable balloon. **B** De Pezzer and **C** Malecot catheters, both inserted after stretching over an introducer. **D** Winsbury White catheter, inserted with the end folded.

A   **B**   **C**

Fig. 4.12 Using a soft, flexible T-tube as a self-retaining catheter. In **A**, it is being inserted through a side hole into the duct. In **B**, the short limb of the 'T' lies in the lumen. It does not obstruct the lumen and allows contents to pass through it or into the long limb. **C** Traction causes the short limbs to come together in order to be pulled out. Any leak rapidly dries up.

in the duct and allows fluid to flow through it or out of the long limb. When the tube is to be removed, apply gentle traction on the long limb and the flexible cross-pieces of the short limb fold together so that it can be pulled out. The minor leakage dries up rapidly unless there is distal obstruction, and this can be excluded beforehand by radiology following injection of contrast medium.

The ability to mould curves in plastic tubes creates a simple means of retaining them. Introduce a pigtailed catheter after first inserting into it a straight guidewire; withdraw the guidewire, enabling it to regain its natural shape. A double pigtailed catheter (Fig. 4.13), resists

movement in either direction, yet when pulled from either end is sufficiently flexible to be withdrawn easily.

Non-self-retaining catheters require some sort of fixation, depending on the circumstances.

1. To retain a catheter indefinitely within a narrow duct, secure it with a ligature or suture–ligature encircling the duct and catheter (Fig. 4.14); the ligature will eventually cut through the wall of the duct. It is difficult to retain a small catheter within the cut end of a wide-bore duct while preventing leakage; try entering the catheter at one side then close the remaining duct lumen with stitches.

2. Catheters emerging through the skin can be fixed to prevent them from being dislodged in a number of ways (Fig. 4.15). Adhesive plaster or tape may suffice. A stitch inserted through the skin and the tube is a secure method but allows leakage through the stitch hole in the tube. Alternatively, place a stitch through the skin and then lace it back and forth around

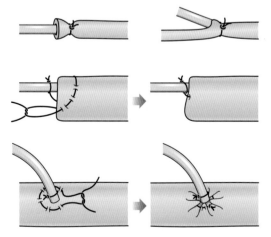

Fig. 4.13 A double pigtailed catheter lies in the ureter. One end is curled in the pelvis of the ureter, the other is curled in the bladder. It may be retrieved easily after grasping the tip within the bladder through a cystoscope.

Fig. 4.14 Fixing catheters into small ducts. At the top on the left the catheter has been inserted into the end of a duct, on the right it is passed through the side, thus retaining the flow through the duct. Below are shown methods needed for fixing them into the end or side of larger ducts.

55

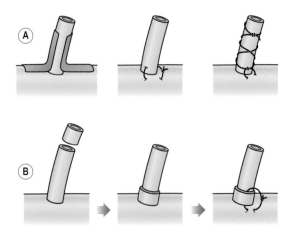

Fig. 4.15 A Methods of fixing catheters to the skin using adhesive plaster or stitches. B Method suggested by Miss Phyllis George: cut a collar from the end of the duct, slip it over the duct and insert a stitch between it and the duct to stitch it to the skin.

Fig. 4.16 Bougies. A Tapered. B Olivary-tipped. C Stepped. D Multiple olives. E Curved rigid. F Malleable. G Hollow dilator threaded over flexible guidewire.

the tube – so-called 'English lacing', after the manner in which the ancient Britons wrapped their lower legs.

3. An elastic catheter can be neatly fixed by a method shown me by my colleague Miss Phyllis George; cut a small segment from the open end of the tube and stretch it to fit over the emerging catheter. Insert a skin stitch incorporating the cuff that does not pierce the emerging catheter.

DILATING DUCTS

Bougies

Bougies (F = candle, from the town in Algeria where they were made) are usually rods or tubes of circular cross-section (Fig. 4.16) with expanded sections that dilate the channel through which they pass. They may be of rigid or malleable metal or semi-rigid plastic. Dilators may be straight or curved. Metal instruments introduced into the urethra or uterus to probe or dilate the passage are often termed 'sounds' (F *sonder* = to prove, to try).

1. Rigid instruments are damaging in clumsy hands but, when used skilfully, give a better 'feel' and the direction can be controlled. Malleable instruments are useful if the shape of the track is irregular.
2. The tip of a dilator is rounded and of smaller diameter than the shank, the transition being gradual. Once the tip has entered the stricture, advancing the instrument gradually dilates it. An olivary-tipped dilator has an oval globular end, likened to an olive; as the olive slips through the stricture its onward passage suddenly becomes easier, providing an estimate of the length of

the narrowing – confirmed if necessary by withdrawing it again and noting when the grip of the stricture is suddenly relaxed. The freedom of the dilator after the olive has passed though the narrowing allows you to retain the 'feel' of the passage beyond. As you advance the dilator, it gradually expands the lumen.

3. Start with the largest dilator that is likely to pass, especially if you are using a rigid instrument, since fine rigid instruments too easily perforate the walls of the channel, which may be diseased and fragile.
4. When appropriate, apply a sterile lubricant such as liquid paraffin or a water-soluble jelly.
5. If possible straighten the channel by exerting traction so there is minimal friction with the walls and you do not lose the 'feel' of the tip. This is possible when you dilate the male urethra.
6. Try varying the direction of the tip until it engages; if this fails, try successively smaller instruments.
7. Multiple strictures require great sensitivity of touch to negotiate them. The grip of each stricture or of a tight orifice dulls your sense of 'feel' for the tip within the next stricture. For this reason dilate each stricture as far as possible before tackling the next one, so that the dilator lies freely until it is gripped by the new stricture.
8. When the tip of the dilator is forcefully pushed through the wall of the channel it creates a space which may become epithelialized, remaining as a diverticulum which a future dilator may enter as a false passage. At subsequent attempts at dilatation the tip of the dilator easily enters into this side channel keeping it open. In the urethra such passages usually develop just distal to a stricture, so you encounter them instead of entering the stricture.

Key points

- You are nearly always dilating a duct because it is strictured, or is blocked by inflammatory swelling or abnormal content.
- If you encounter resistance or bleeding there is a reason.
- Your likeliest way of determining the cause is to hold the dilator with your fingertips and 'feel' the obstructing surface as you gently probe it.

9. Withdraw the dilator and advance it once more while you keep the tip pressed against the opposite wall. It is suggested that one dilator can be left in the false passage to block its mouth while a second instrument passes along the main duct. I have never succeeded with this method.

10. A filiform (L *filum* = thread, hence threadlike) flexible bougie may be induced to follow a tortuous path through the stricture. If it passes through, a dilator can be screwed to it and guided by it through the stricture; the flexibility of the filiform leader allows it to fold upon itself within a cavity beyond the stricture (Fig. 4.17), where it can be captured, drawn through with a dilator attached to follow its path.

11. *Seldinger's wire* (see Ch. 5) is a useful method of following a tortuous channel and negotiating a difficult stricture. Pass the flexible tipped guidewire through the stricture by gently rotating it back and forth as you advance it through the stricture. Radiographic monitoring of the progress of the tip of the radio-opaque guidewire is invaluable. You may be able to introduce contrast medium to outline the passage. When you have succeeded in advancing the guidewire through the stricture, thread over it a close-fitting but not tight dilator which has a central hole and gently advance this down to and through the stricture (Fig. 4.16G). At intervals ensure that the guidewire moves freely within the dilator; fixation of the guidewire indicates that it is trapped and kinked so the tip of the dilator is not entering the stricture and could perforate the side wall of the duct.

12. *Endoscopic guidance*, when available, allows you to visualize one end of the stricture so that you are able to negotiate a guidewire through it under vision, as in the oesophagus. You can leave the guidewire in place, remove the endoscope and pass graded dilators that have a central channel over the guidewire to dilate the stricture.

13. Occasionally it is impossible to pass even a fine guidewire through. In some circumstances, if one end of a thread is fixed proximally and the other end is introduced above the stricture, this will eventually be carried through by fluid flow and by peristalsis. After retrieving the distal end, attach a thin, flexible dilator to the proximal end. Exert slight traction on the distal thread to guide and draw through the tip of the fine dilator (Fig. 4.18). I have used this method (devised by Mr Richard Franklin), using the radio-opaque marker thread of a surgical swab as a leader, with success in overcoming seemingly impassable oesophageal strictures.

14. Commonly, you can pass a series of graduated dilators, each one being slightly thicker than the previous one. As you negotiate the stricture, note the details of the passage. Do not remove it until you have the next dilator ready. Now smoothly draw out the first dilator and immediately and gently slide in the next size, and so on. The tip of each bigger dilator is slightly smaller than the shank of its predecessor. Control the direction of insertion and passage of a rigid dilator by movement of the handle (Fig. 4.19). A rigid curved dilator cannot be rotated while it lies in a narrow channel but if it reaches a wider channel it can be rotated. Confirm that you have reached the bladder by this method when dilating urethral strictures.

15. Occasionally you may need to stretch a normal channel very gently, in order to insert instruments or substances, for example the meatus and penile urethra, to pass a large instrument such as a prostatic resectoscope.

Fig. 4.17 Using a filiform leader as a pilot for the dilator.

Fig. 4.18 A thread has been induced to pass the stricture and acts as a leader for the dilator.

Key points

- Do not be too ambitious – be willing to stop before you achieve the maximum diameter, and repeat the procedure at increasing intervals, gaining a little each time.
- If you overstretch it and split the lining, usually signalled by bleeding, the stricture will recur.
- Never fail to record the size of the dilators and details of the peculiarities of the passage on each occasion, for future guidance.

Fig. 4.20 The catheter carries a collapsed balloon, which can be placed within a stricture. When the balloon is inflated it exerts a radial dilating effect.

Fig. 4.19 Negotiating a curved channel with a rigid curved dilator. The handle of the dilator must be swung in an arc to direct the point along the curved path.

Balloons

When a dilator is pushed through a stricture there is a damaging shear force on the duct lining. As this heals, scar tissue is laid down, which contracts as it matures, recreating the stricture. When possible, avoid the shearing force by exerting centrifugal distension only, from within the stricture. An excellent method of achieving this is by balloon dilatation. Over-distension of the balloon may disrupt the wall; for this reason balloons are available that reach a predetermined maximum diameter or pressure then rupture if over-inflated.

1. Negotiate a collapsed balloon across the stricture and inflate it, exerting only radial forces (Fig. 4.20). The balloons can be passed under vision, mounted on catheters threaded over guidewires, or over endoscopes. They can be accurately placed under radiological control and for this reason they usually incorporate radio-opaque markers at each end of the balloon.
2. Balloon dilatation is sometimes used to overstretch the sphincteric muscles of, for example, the lower oesophagus to overcome a hold-up resulting from achalasia (G *a* = not + *chalasis* = relaxation) – failure to relax as a bolus of food reaches it to pass through into the stomach.

Other methods

1. Dilators that expand while they lie within a narrow channel have been used for many years. A classic method is a laminaria tent (L *tenta* = a probe) in which a cylinder of dried seaweed is inserted in a duct; as it absorbs water it expands and dilates the channel. The method has long been in use to dilate the uterine cervical canal to procure an abortion.
2. Mechanical expansile dilatation from within the lumen was devised to dilate stenosed heart valves.
3. *Stents*, named after the English dentist Charles Stent (1807–1885), are increasingly used to hold open passages that have been dilated. One type can be sited as a long, narrow tube within a stricture and then expanded by inflating a balloon within it, expanding the stent which then retains its shape, preventing restenosis.
4. Special materials have been developed in the last few years in order to produce wire mesh elastic self-expanding stents. The mesh is compressed to produce a long thin tube that is released when it lies across the narrowing. It actively adopts a shorter and wider shape that progressively expands the narrowed segment.
5. When the lumen of a duct is encroached on by an ingrowth of diseased tissue such as cancer, the passage can often be restored using several forms of treatment including diathermy, radiotherapy, laser therapy and chemotherapy. Photodynamic treatment of certain tumours consists of giving a sensitizing agent which is taken up by the encroaching cells, then using laser light to produce selective tumour cell necrosis.

ENDOSCOPIC ACCESS

1. Endoscopy (G *endon* = within + *skopein* = to view) and 'down the line of sight' operative procedures have been well established for many years through an extensive range of rigid and flexible endoscopes. Instruments can be inserted into natural tubes and

manoeuvred by 'feel'. Advances were possible because of improvements in visualization and instrumentation. Improvements in imaging reduce the need for physical exploration.

2. A wide range of instruments can be introduced through open tubes or through special channels in more sophisticated endoscopes with good lighting and visual characteristics, into natural or abnormal channels, including catheters, dilators, balloons, diathermy wires, forceps, scissors, cytology brushes, Dormia baskets and snares (Fig. 4.21). These may be rigid or flexible and controllable.

3. Instruments with moving parts such as scissors, forceps and snares can be activated by two rods sliding on each other, or one rod sliding within a rigid tube; the moving rod can be pushed or pulled. Flexible instruments often employ the principle attributed to Sir Frank Bowden (circa 1902, founder of Raleigh bicycles, for the brake cables). The inner wire can be pulled but not pushed within the outer flexible tube; if the inner wire has been pulled, release must be by some distal spring action. Handle designs vary but all rely on a gripping motion or separation of the hand or of a finger and thumb (Fig. 4.22). Because the tissues cannot be held and steadied while they are being cut with scissors, the blades may

advantageously be claw-shaped (Fig. 4.21), to prevent the tissue from sliding away.

4. When introducing a rigid instrument along a convoluted channel, be extremely sensitive to the hold-ups. Be willing to withdraw it slightly, adjust the angle and gently advance it again. Try to keep the tip of the instrument in the centre of the lumen.

5. If a straight instrument has an angled tip it may be rotated within a flexible but twisting channel to assist the progress of its tip. A classic example is the shape of a rigid cystoscope for passage through the male urethra. Once the angled tip of the cystoscope enters the bladder cavity it can be rotated and moved – the shaft has straightened the urethra (Fig. 4.23). Although cystoscopy is now generally performed with a flexible instrument there are occasions when only a rigid instrument may be available or suitable.

6. Of necessity, rigid instruments passed under vision must be manoeuvred along the line of sight. Depth perception is limited. The point of action of instruments with an offset tip can be controlled by rotating them.

7. Flexible instruments are difficult to control within a wide channel or open tube but their flexibility may facilitate progression along a tortuous track. However, the tip may engage in an irregularity; if it does,

Fig. 4.21 Some of the instruments that can be used down an endoscope. **A** Catheter. **B** Dilator. **C** Diathermy wire tightened to produce a 'cheese-cutter' effect. **D** Forceps. **E** Scissors. **F** Cytology brush. **G** Dormier basket. **H** A snare.

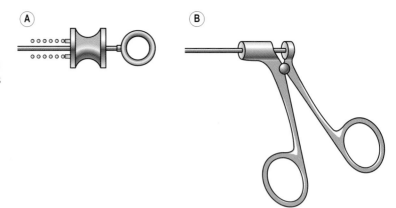

Fig. 4.22 Methods of controlling moving tipped instruments. **A** A wire passes through a spiral wire flexible tube. This Bowden cable mechanism can be pulled but not pushed. **B** A rigid system of a rod passing through a metal tube. This allows both pulling and pushing.

Fig. 4.23 A bent but flexible duct such as a male urethra can be straightened. The angled tip of the instrument follows the bends of the urethra because it can be rotated. Once it enters the bladder the tip can be freely rotated and advanced or withdrawn.

Fig. 4.24 A flexible catheter or instrument can be passed out of the side of a rigid or flexible endoscope. The angle of emergence can be controlled using an Albarran lever.

withdraw it slightly, rotate it and gently advance it. Remember, there is less 'feel' with a flexible instrument than with a rigid one.

8. An instrument or catheter can be led out of a tube through a side hole to angulate it (Fig. 4.24). Some rigid and flexible endoscopes have a controllable lever to vary the angle of emergence. This was originally designed by the Parisian urologist of Cuban origin, Jacques Albarran (1860–1912). The tip of the instrument or tube can be kept in view through a side-viewing telescope.

Rigid instruments

The cystoscope was the first endoscopic instrument to reach a very high standard of development. Through it, you may inspect the bladder, take biopsies, fulgurate tumours and catheterize ureters. Fibreoptic cystoscopes can be passed relatively painlessly. Urethroscopy, ureteroscopy and percutaneous nephrostomy can be carried out. Transurethral resection of the prostate gland can be achieved using a diathermy loop, through a resectoscope.

Sigmoidoscopy is now usually carried out using a flexible instrument but you may need, because of the circumstances, to use a rigid instrument. Take the opportunity to practise gentle, skilful manipulation of a tube.

1. Place the patient on the left side, buttocks overhanging the right side of the couch, knees drawn up to the chest, feet on the far side from you as you stand on the right side of the couch (Fig. 4.25).

> **Key point**
>
> • Never insert an endoscope without first inspecting the peri-anal area and carrying out a careful digital examination, after explaining to the patient what you are doing.

2. Gently place the tip of the obturator within the well-lubricated sigmoidoscope (Fig. 4.26) against the patient's anus, pointing towards the umbilicus. Maintain only slight pressure until the sphincter relaxes, allowing you to insert the sigmoidoscope for about 6–8 cm when it abuts against the anterior wall of the rectum. Hold the sigmoidoscope steady while you withdraw the obturator and fit on the viewing end seal with attached light bulb and air pump.
3. Perform all subsequent manoeuvres under vision. Insufflate only sufficient air to separate the walls and allow you to guide the endoscope safely without

Fig. 4.25 Sigmoidoscopy, seen from above. The sigmoidoscope is angled after initial insertion to view the rectum, which lies in the hollow of the sacrum.

Battery

Fig. 4.26 A A short proctoscope, which is an open hollow tube. The obturator has been withdrawn. **B** A rigid sigmoidoscope, which is an open tube that can be closed off so the bowel can be inflated and distended. The cap has a transparent window.

causing discomfort. You are now close up to the anterior rectal wall. To regain the view of the lumen you need to swing the outer end of the endoscope anteriorly to turn the internal portion into the rectum lying in the hollow of the sacrum. Concentrate initially on introducing the instrument

to the intended limit, keeping the tip centred in the bowel lumen. As you withdraw it in a spiral manner you can examine every part of the interior, paying particular attention to the mucosa and any abnormalities.

4. If you wish to remove a biopsy or swab specimen, you must remove the viewing end and allow the air to escape. First of all bring into the centre of view your objective; usually you can trap it by enclosing it and gently pressing the tip of the instrument against the bowel wall. Do not over-inflate the rectum or it will suddenly deflate and the target mucosa will move. Insert the biopsy forceps or swab, and obtain the specimen, then replace the viewing end-piece so that you can reinflate the rectum and complete the examination.

5. Deflate the rectum and warn the patient as you finally withdraw the sigmoidoscope, since it feels like an embarrassing defecation.

Proctoscopy is carried out in a similar manner but retain the obturator until you have fully introduced the instrument. Once more, remember that you must swing the handle portion forward on the patient to negotiate the almost 90° angle between anus and rectum. Only now should you remove the obturator.

1. Carefully view the interior of the lower rectum and anal canal as you slowly withdraw the proctoscope.

2. As the rim of the proctoscope descends in the anal canal, the sphincter attempts to extrude it and you need to apply slight counter pressure to prevent this while you examine the lower anal canal.

61

Haemorrhoid injection with sclerosant must be made into the perivascular tissues around the upper pole of each pile.

1. During your first introduction and withdrawal of the proctoscope take careful note of the situation of the haemorrhoids as they prolapse over the lip of the withdrawing endoscope. Traditionally they were recorded as though the patient lay supine in the lithotomy position at 4, 7 and 11 o'clock related to a clock face. Since the patient now usually lies on the left side, they are usually at 1, 4 and 8 o'clock.

2. As you withdraw the proctoscope until the piles prolapse into the lumen, they obscure your view of their bases. You must now remove the proctoscope, replace the obturator, fully reintroduce it and again remove the obturator to inject at the base of each haemorrhoid.

3. Slowly withdraw the proctoscope until a rim of anus appears, and the sphincter begins to extrude the proctoscope. Resist this but angle the proctoscope to reveal a complete ring of about 0.5 cm of anal canal. If the haemorrhoids prolapse you are too low; withdraw the proctoscope, reinsert it and start again.

4. Taking each site in turn, insert the shouldered needle attached to the filled haemorrhoid syringe. Aspirate. If blood enters the syringe you are within the vessel. Fully withdraw the needle and reinsert it in a slightly different site until you cannot aspirate any blood.

5. Inject approximately 5–10 mL of 5% phenol in almond or arachis (peanut) oil into the submucosa at the base of the pile. Watch as you inject. You should produce a slight swelling; if the swelling blanches, you are too superficial, if there is no swelling you are too deep.

Key points

- Haemorrhoid injection cannot be performed with a single insertion of the proctoscope.
- Injection must be perivascular, into the base of each pile, and never into the vessel.

Other rigid instruments. Laryngoscopes, auriscopes (L *auris* = ear), colposcopes (G *kolpos* = sinus or pocket but applied to the vagina), hysteroscope (G *hysteros* = womb), and many other endoscopes are used. In some cases the instrument is called a speculum (L = a mirror, from *spectare* = to look) since a mirror was inserted. Nasal and vaginal specula are in common use.

Key points

- Safe passage of instruments for the various forms of single access to tubes and spaces, requires specialized training, especially in order to interpret the findings and perform procedures that sometimes demand skills at the limits of technical accomplishment.
- Some procedures, such as laryngoscopy, proctoscopy and sigmoidoscopy, should be well within the capability of any surgical trainee. Take every opportunity to learn how to use these endoscopes safely and effectively.

Flexible endoscopes

Fibreoptic endoscopy became possible following the development of coherent glass fibre bundles by Harold Hopkins (1918–1994) in Reading, UK (Fig. 4.27). Basil Hirschowitz of Birmingham, Alabama improved the fibres and introduced gastrointestinal endoscopy.

A variety of controllable, flexible endoscopes can be passed into the upper and lower gastrointestinal tract (Fig. 4.28), the trachea and bronchi, urinary and gynaeco-logical tracts, and other tubes, blood vessels, joints and tissue spaces. The instruments are remarkably versatile and allow, for example, inspection, biopsy, snaring, dilatation and diathermization, and facilitate the capture, ultrasonic shock and laser beam fragmentation of stones, among other specialized procedures.

Fig. 4.27 A coherent bundle of glass fibres. They transmit light in a constant relationship within the fibres throughout the bundle.

Fig. 4.28 The end of a flexible controllable fibreoptic endoscope. There are two light-carrying ports and one optical port. Top right is a channel for biopsy forceps, cytology brush, catheters and other instruments. Suction, insufflation and lens spraying facilities are also incorporated.

DISPLAY

Some ducts, such as the bowel, lie free while others, such as intrahepatic bile ducts and bronchi, are buried in connective tissue. Take every opportunity to recognize ducts by gaining an intimate knowledge of the anatomy, appearance and feel. For example, the ureter has a characteristic vermiculating peristalsis. Ducts opening onto a surface, such as the urethra and salivary ducts, can be catheterized to delineate their paths. Fistulous tracks can be followed by inserting a probe or injecting dye.

Radio-opaque media can be injected through catheters, administered orally or parenterally and may be secreted or excreted into ducts to be displayed on X-rays, such as cholecystograms and urograms. Other imaging methods may also be used to aid identification and location.

1. When seeking a duct lying in homogeneous tissue, always cut in the expected line of the duct rather than at right angles to it, to avoid the risk of transecting it.
2. If you wish to display a long segment of duct take care not to damage any tributaries or divisions and respect its blood and nervous supply.
3. Remember that a collapsed and empty duct may be imperceptible, but can be made more prominent by gently distending it with fluid, catheterizing or cannulating it.
4. Protect a fragile duct from injury as you display it by separating overlying tissues with care. Gently insert the rounded tips of non-toothed dissecting forceps superficial to the duct, allow them to open, and cut between the separated blades (Fig. 4.29). Blunt-nosed haemostatic forceps are valuable dissecting instruments when freeing ducts; insinuate the closed blades next to the duct and gently open them parallel to the duct (Fig. 4.30). If the duct has tributaries or if it branches, it is sometimes preferable to open the forceps at right angles to the duct (Fig. 4.31).

Fig. 4.29 Display a duct by placing dissecting forceps superficial to it, allow the forceps blades to separate, and cut between them.

Fig. 4.30 Displaying a duct by opening haemostatic forceps parallel to it.

Fig. 4.31 Displaying a duct by opening haemostatic forceps at right angles to it.

5. It may be possible to inject methylene blue dye into a duct, such as a thyroglossal fistula, so that if it is inadvertently entered or transected, dye leaks out to warn you – but in my hands it has usually leaked and caused general staining. Another method is to pass in a probe or catheter; for example, the ureter can be catheterized through a cystoscope if you need to preserve it from injury when subsequently dissecting structures nearby in difficult circumstances.

OCCLUSION

Divided duct

1. The duct may be divided deliberately or accidentally.
2. Diathermization under compression creates a weld in a small duct but check that it has been effective. Ultrasonic welding is an alternative method of closure (see Ch. 2).

3. If it is important that the channel does not reform, as when carrying out vasectomy or female sterilization by occluding the fallopian tubes, divide them after doubly ligating or clipping them and separate the ends.
4. Ligation is usually safe and effective but do not tie it too tightly or it may cut right through. Do not apply the ligature too near the end or it may slip off or be gradually rolled off if the duct undergoes peristalsis (Fig. 4.32). As a safeguard against this, insert a transfixion suture–ligature (Fig. 4.33). If spillage of contents is a risk, apply double ligatures before transecting the duct between them (Fig 4.34).
5. Close a supple large-bore duct using a simple ligature reinforced by invaginating the end within a purse-string suture (Fig. 4.35).
6. Flatten a supple but thicker-walled duct and close it with a linear suture (Fig. 4.36). This can be reinforced by invaginating it within a second layer of sutures (Fig. 4.37).
7. A single metal, or absorbable clip is sufficient to occlude a small duct. Close the flattened end of a larger duct with a linear stapler (Fig. 4.38).

Key point

- When there is a choice, prefer sutures to clips; they are more versatile – and less likely to catch in other tissues, instruments or materials, and be dragged off.

Fig. 4.32 Do not apply ligatures too near the end of a duct. The one on the right may slip off or be rolled off by peristalsis.

Fig. 4.33 Transfixion suture–ligature. The needled thread has been passed through the duct before being tied.

Fig. 4.34 If there is a risk of spillage, do not transect the duct until you have applied two ligatures at a distance from each other, then cut between them.

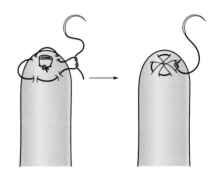

Fig. 4.35 On the left a ligature has been tied to close the end of a large duct. On the right the closed end has been invaginated with a purse-string suture.

Fig. 4.36 Closing a wide-bore tube with a row of sutures after flattening the end.

In continuity

If you wish to occlude a small supple duct without dividing it, apply a ligature, or a metal clip. Larger supple tubes cannot be occluded in this manner and must be flattened and closed with a line of stitches or a line of staples.

Control of leakage

1. Achieve temporary control of an actual or potential leak from a duct by simple compression, constriction with a thread or tape ligature, or apply one of the

Fig. 4.37 A linear suture-closure (or staple-closure) of a duct can be reinforced by invaginating the first suture line with a second layer of sutures.

(A)

(B)

Fig. 4.38 Closing a deformable tube with a double row of staples. **A** Apply the stapler across the duct and actuate it. **B** When the stapler is removed the double line of staples can be seen.

Fig. 4.39 The curved Satinsky-type clamp allows flow along the lower part of the duct as the open upper part is isolated to control leakage.

Fig. 4.40 The tube has an external cuff that can be inflated through a side tube. This channels all fluids through the tube lumen. The technique facilitates inflation of the lungs through a cuffed endotracheal tube (see Fig. 4.8).

DISOBLITERATION

A duct can be blocked as a result of many factors or a combination:

Intraluminal: the contents, for example inspissated (L *spissare* = thicken) contents, worms, flukes in the bowel, stones in the ureter, bile duct or salivary duct, polyps and various foods or bezoars (Persian – ingested concretions), block the lumen.

Intramural: (L *murus* = wall) such as a stricture, tumour, or failure to transmit the contents by peristalsis. The presence of a tumour in the wall of the intestine may obstruct the passage by blocking the lumen or, by its rigidity, stop the run of peristaltic waves – often generating the classical 'change of bowel habit'.

Extramural: external factors as from adhesions, bands, hernial orifices and external tumours.

> ### Key points
>
> - How you manage the blockage depends upon its cause – is it likely to recur?
> - If the cause is progressive, for example malignant obstruction, you need to isolate any corrective procedure from encroachment by the disease.

large variety of non-crushing clamps to occlude the flow of content upstream of the site of the leak. The curved Satinsky-type clamp does not obstruct flow along the duct but isolates a potential source of leakage while it is being repaired, joined or closed (Fig. 4.39).

2. Alternatively, occlude the lumen using a balloon obturator such as a Foley catheter, which can be deflated and withdrawn at the last minute before final closure. If necessary, fluid can be introduced into, or drained from the duct through the main channel of the catheter.

3. The principle of a cuffed tube is employed when an endotracheal tube is passed to inflate the lungs during anaesthesia or to provide respiratory assistance (Fig. 4.40). Inflate the cuff, lying in the trachea, to prevent leakage around the tube during respiratory inflation.

1. If obstruction results from a stricture it may be dilated. A tumour can be shrunk by external radiotherapy, local irradiation – brachytherapy (G *brachys* = short, short range), or chemotherapy.
2. Stones can often be pulverized (L *pulvis* = powder) by shock-wave lithotripsy (G *lithos* = stone + *ripsis* = rubbing), ultrasound or laser therapy. Accessible stones can be crushed, and with other obstructions, can often be removed using forceps or other instruments passed through an endoscope (Fig. 4.41). In some cases disobliteration can be carried out endoscopically either by excision, as in diathermy loop transurethral resection of the prostate, or by vaporization with a laser beam, as with oesophageal carcinoma.
3. The lumen can often be restored by inserting a splinting tube (Fig. 4.42). This may be placed after first dilating the narrow segment and leaving in a bougie, then passing over this a plastic tube advanced through the narrow segment with a 'pusher' tube (Fig. 4.43). Insertion of such tubes often demands immediate and extensive preliminary dilatation. In many sites this can be avoided by inserting a tube stent made of springy metal that can be introduced across the narrowing in a compressed state and allowed to expand spontaneously (Fig. 4.44).
4. It may be necessary to deal with an obstruction by open operation. On occasion non-invasive methods have failed, or are inappropriate. For example, normal or diseased bowel may be obstructed by a

Key points

- Inserting a stent into a tube or duct that normally passes on the contents by peristalsis creates an aperistaltic segment.
- Transmission is seriously prejudiced and viscous or solid contents may obstruct within the stent.

Fig. 4.42 A plastic hollow stent has been impacted in a tube to hold it open. The flared upper end is designed to prevent the stent from passing through the stricture.

Fig. 4.43 The safest way to introduce a stent is to dilate the stricture and leave a bougie within the lumen. Slide the stent over the bougie, using a 'pusher', to advance it into position, then remove the pusher and bougie.

Fig. 4.41 Instruments for removing obstructions. **A** A rigid 'alligator' forceps. **B** and **C** Flexible grasping forceps, shown closed and open. **D** A Dormier basket, shown closed and open. **E** A balloon catheter, shown deflated and inflated. **F** An internal ring stripper.

swallowed foreign body, impacted food, a gall-stone that has ulcerated into the bowel, or a ball of intestinal worms. Do not immediately open the duct. Soft material may be disimpacted, broken up and manoeuvred through a narrow segment and allowed to pass through normally. If this is

Fig. 4.44 Expanding stent. The springy wire stent is compressed, making it long and thin. When it is correctly placed across the stricture it is released and expands its diameter while shortening its length, expanding the narrow segment.

impossible, consider massaging it proximally and open the duct where the wall is less likely to have suffered damage. Remove the cause of the block and carefully repair the opening. This is now rarely required for impacted stones in the ureter, bile ducts or salivary ducts. Especially when removing salivary duct stones guard against them slipping back into the gland by encircling the duct with a thread or a gently closed tissue forceps, before opening the duct (Fig. 4.45).

5. Obstruction of the bowel commonly results from pressure or kinking by adhesions – originally fibrinous, often becoming fibrous strands, usually but not always resulting from a previous inflammation or an operation. A second cause is herniation in which the intestine protrudes through a restricted hole within which the entrapped bowel becomes blocked. Infrequently, bowel is blocked by spontaneous twisting, and also by intussusception in which the bowel draws itself within the lumen and passes it along.

6. A narrow segment of a supple duct can be widened by a plastic (G *plassein* = to form) procedure. It was originally devised to overcome strictures resulting from long-standing ulceration at the pylorus and named **pyloroplasty**. It has been adapted for dealing with the small bowel strictures resulting from *Crohn's inflammatory bowel disease*. Make a longitudinal incision through the full length of the stricture, open it out and close the defect as a transverse suture line (Fig. 4.46).

7. It may be preferable to excise a narrow segment and bring the ends together directly to bridge the defect (Fig 4.47A). The circumferential suture line that results may narrow the lumen; if so, minimize this by cutting the duct diagonally at each end of the stricture, producing a longer oblique line of closure (Fig. 4.47B).

8. *Immovable or recurrent obstruction* can be dealt with in many ways. You may accept the blockage; an example is blockage of a ureter below a poorly functioning kidney with good function of the other kidney. One method of relief is bypass, creating an internal stoma (G = mouth) with the duct below the obstruction or with another channel, for example

Fig. 4.46 Overcome a longitudinal stricture with an incision along its whole length. Open it out, draw the two ends of the incision together and close the defect as a transverse incision, creating a shorter but wider tube.

Fig. 4.45 Removing an obstructing stone from a superficial duct. A stitch prevents the stone from escaping proximally. In **A**, the stone is near the orifice, which can be opened up with scissors to release the stone. In **B**, the stone lies some distance from the orifice. Cut down onto the stone through the overlying epithelium, leaving the duct orifice intact. Pull the thread through after removing the stone.

Fig. 4.47 A Excise the stricture and join the cut ends. **B** End-to-end anastomosis with a circumferential suture line may leave a constriction. This can be avoided by cutting the ends obliquely and joining them.

draining a blocked bile duct or ureter into the bowel. A duct that is merely a transmitter, not secreting any substance into the lumen, may be divided above and below the obstruction, with the proximal and distal cut ends united; an irremovable obstructed segment is left in situ. In the case of, for example, the bowel, which secretes substances such as mucus, an irremovable segment cannot usually be left undrained. The creation of an *external stoma* may be valuable because it not only clears the secretion but also allows the output to be measured.

Key points

- Differentiate between a duct that is merely a conduit and one that secretes or fills with content; for example, the bowel secretes enzymes and mucus.
- If the duct secretes into the lumen, you must not leave a closed segment or loop which will become distended with its own secretions.

---

9. Methods of bypass are shown in Fig. 4.48. It may be possible without transecting the duct (Fig. 4.48A1). Draw up a distal loop proximally and unite it above the obstruction, to carry on the obstructed contents (Fig. 4.48A2). Contents may stagnate in the segment between the obstruction and the stoma. An external stoma can also be created without transecting the duct (Fig. 4.48A3); again, content may stagnate in the segment between the obstruction and the external stoma.

   The duct may be transected below the obstruction (Fig. 4.48B1), allowing you to draw up the distal cut end above it (Fig. 4.48B2), and close off the stump below the obstruction. Do not close off the stump if it is likely to become

distended; prefer to join the cut end into the draining loop (Fig. 4.48B3), or bring it to the surface (Fig. 4.48B4); this is often termed a draining fistula (L = pipe) to distinguish it from a stoma that drains the whole duct content.

The duct may be transected above an irremovable obstruction (Fig. 4.48C1) and brought to the surface as a stoma (Fig. 4.48C2). If a secreting remnant above the obstruction is closed off, it may become filled and rupture. One solution is to create a loop stoma (Fig. 4.48A3) but to prevent any flow down the loop, separate stomas can be created (Fig. 4.48C3), so the proximal duct is drained but also the duct between the distal cut end and the obstruction. If you cannot drain the segment internally or bring it to the surface as a stoma, consider inserting a tube to bridge the distance between the loop and the surface (Fig. 4.49). If the tube points upwards it tends to drain downwards and can be collected into a bag. If it points downwards, the contents may need to be sucked out. If the tube remains in position for a considerable period, a fistulous track may form so that the contents reach the surface even when the tube is withdrawn.

10. *Strangulation* (G *strangos* = twisted) implies cutting off the blood supply by twisting or by constriction, as may occur in herniation of bowel through a rigid orifice. Content may flow in but if outflow is restricted the bowel distends and is liable to become irreducible. Inflow at arterial pressure in the presence of venous compression and restricted outflow causes vascular congestion, stagnation, capillary distension, rupture and extravasation. At this stage the bowel is still viable but appears black, like a bruise, the serosa is shiny, the arterial pulse is still palpable but of course the subserosal haematoma will take many days to be reabsorbed. If the bowel is not released the arterial inflow ceases and anoxic blood stagnates. The mucosa, which is the most metabolically active part, begins to die and bacteria, flourishing in the lumen, pass through it as gangrene spreads through the wall. The serosal sheen is lost as the colour changes to grey and green. Colic continues in the bowel above but there is a continuous underlying pain and tenderness.

Key points

- Recognize incipient strangulation.
- Urgently release and if necessary resect strangulated bowel.

REPAIR

Ducts may be damaged accidentally or deliberately – as when performing a surgical manoeuvre to gain access or as part of a radical resection of spreading disease.

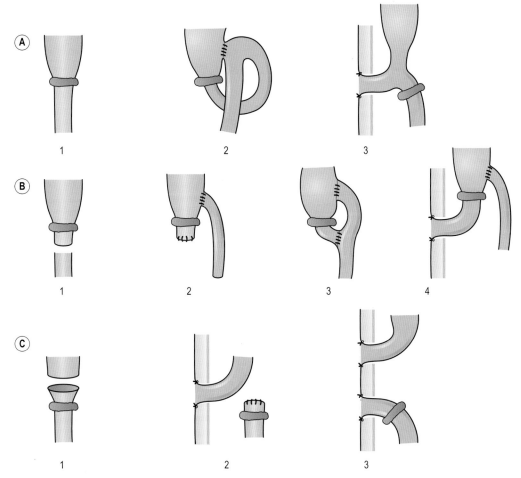

Fig. 4.48 Possibilities for dealing with an irremovable obstruction. **A (1)** Do not transect the obstructed segment above or below the blockage. **(2)** Draw up a distal loop from beyond the obstruction and form an anastomosis proximal to the obstruction. **(3)** Bring the segment above the obstruction to the surface to form an external stoma. **B (1)** Transect the distal duct below the obstruction. **(2)** Draw the lower cut end proximally to unite it above the obstruction. Close off the distal stump beyond the block. **(3)** If there is a risk of the remnant below becoming distended by local secretions if it is closed, join it into the draining loop or **(4)** bring it to the surface as a draining fistula. **C (1)** Transect the bowel above the obstruction. **(2)** Bring out the upper cut end to the surface as a terminal stoma and close the stump above the block. **(3)** If the closed stump is likely to become distended, bring the stump to the surface as a draining fistula.

Fig. 4.49 If you need to leave a fixed, closed compartment that may fill up, and which cannot be drained internally, insert a self-retaining catheter. Bring the catheter to the exterior. A drain inserted upwards can be connected to a bag for collection but one inserted downwards may require suction drainage.

> **Key point**
>
> - To achieve success, carry out the repair perfectly, without tension, on a healthy duct with an adequate blood supply and protect it during the healing phase.

Gastrointestinal tract

1. If the bowel has been injured, assiduously search for every possible blunt or penetrating wound. Check the mesentery for potential threats to the blood supply.
2. The area of the folded mucosa is far greater than the area of the submucosa and seromuscularis, particularly in the small intestine. When the bowel wall is acutely breached, therefore, the mucosa tends to evert. This brings into apposition the mucosal surfaces, forming a channel for leakage of contents (Fig. 4.50). If it is difficult to replace the mucosa, use an inverting mattress stitch, often referred to in this context as a Connell stitch, after the 19th-century American surgeon who popularized it.
3. In contrast, a breach resulting from chronic ulceration or inflammation is associated with fibrosis that fixes the mucosa, so that it does not protrude. As a rule you can safely bring the margins together with a simple all-coats suture as in closing a *perforated peptic ulcer*, although many surgeons include an overlying tag of omentum in the closing stitch.
4. In some cases a large, chronic, rigid, adherent ulcer cannot be closed. A leaked anastomosis will often break down again if you attempt to close it. In both cases it is safer to insert a catheter into the hole and drain it to the surface. A track will form and when you remove the catheter, the hole will close – provided there is no distal obstruction! Occasionally you can deal with the problem by diverting the bowel content to prevent it from reaching the defect, either by creating a proximal stoma or by forming an anastomosis proximal to the defect.

Other ducts and cavities

1. Because many ducts are of small calibre, repair of defects or injuries may result in a stricture; this becomes more likely if you fail to appose the lining epithelium with every stitch. Carefully excise all necrotic tissue or the repair will break down. In many cases the best option is re-anastomosis or anastomosis to a large duct such as bowel.
2. Recognize iatrogenic (G *iatros* = physician) injuries and repair them immediately, especially bile ducts and ureter. The pancreatic duct is not usually repaired but drained into the bowel.

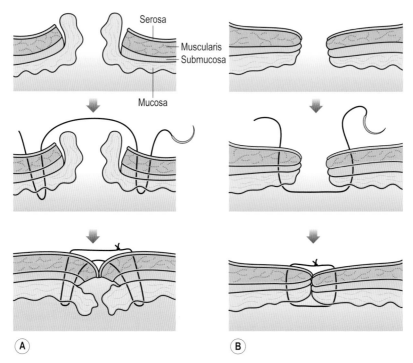

Fig. 4.50 Repair of traumatic rupture of bowel. **A** Section through an acute traumatic puncture of the bowel wall often results in pouting of the mucosa; this can be corrected using an inverting (Connell) mattress suture. **B** A chronic cause has resulted in fibrosis with fixation of the layers; it can be closed using a simple stitch, producing an edge-to-edge union.

3. Repair of the ovarian tubes, vas deferens, salivary and lachrymal ducts demands microsurgical methods (see Ch. 5), in order to preserve or regain tubal patency.

4. Repair of a cavity wall, such as the urinary bladder, is less critical because there is more available tissue. Urologists usually employ stitches that exclude the mucosa – extramucosal stitches. The bladder can contract very powerfully, so it is usual to insert a suprapubic or transurethral catheter to ensure that pressure does not build up.

RESECTION

Bowel needs to be resected without leaking of contents, so crushing clamps are placed across the ends of the segment to be excised, which seals them. You must doubly ligate and divide blood vessels supplying the segment in the mesentery, sometimes recreating the mesentery of bowel, which is described as retro-mesenteric; in fact the mesentery has fused with the posterior parietal peritoneum. You may need to repair the mesentery following resection.

Other ducts. Take great care, when mobilizing small ducts, not to damage the blood supply, which is often tenuous (L *tenuis* = thin). For this reason do not try to free it excessively. In some cases the adventitia – the loose tissue surrounding the duct – carries small vessels and the duct is deprived if this tissue is stripped off. Autonomic nerves, which carry motor impulses to peristaltic muscle and also have an important trophic impulses effect, are also stripped off. Make certain the repair will not narrow the duct and cause obstruction.

ANASTOMOSIS

Galen (AD 131–201) used this term (G *ana* = through + *stoma* = a mouth, hence a coming together through a mouth). Ducts of the same or different types can be joined together.

Principles

1. Ducts of all types must retain or gain an adequate arterial blood supply and venous drainage, in order to heal.
2. Ensure that the anastomosis is performed between disease-free ducts. Inflammation, infection, neoplasms or foreign bodies all threaten healing.
3. Do not join ducts without excluding distal obstruction.
4. Some ducts, notably the bowel, have autonomous directional peristalsis. If you forget this, drainage of the contents may be impaired.

5. Ensure that there is no tension, no twisting or excessive constriction when ducts are joined.
6. Avoid back pressure and stagnation; bacteria rapidly flourish in stagnant contents.

Bowel

1. Ensure the bowel ends match. If they do not, be willing to angle the end of the narrower end, to enlarge it. Cut back on the edge opposite the entrance of the blood supply – the antimesenteric edge (Fig. 4.51).
2. You may apply non-crushing bowel clamps to steady the ends and prevent leakage of content. Alternatively, insert sutures at each end uniting the ends but clipped instead of tying them – 'stay' or 'traction' sutures (Fig. 4.52). If you need to suture the back wall first when the bowel cannot be rotated, insert the traction sutures just posterior to the junction of the back and front walls, so that the anterior walls remain slack when the sutures are distracted, allowing easy access to the back wall. Some surgeons distract the middle of the anterior walls with traction sutures or tissue forceps to provide the best possible access while they insert stitches in the back wall.
3. Types of stitch are determined by your beliefs, training and current fashion, since no satisfactory controlled trials have been carried out comparing popular methods. The strongest and therefore most important layer to include is the submucous, collagenous coat – the coat from which catgut is made. The traditional stitch takes in all coats (Fig. 4.53), attributed to William Halsted (1852–1922) the great American surgeon. A method that is popular at present is an extramucosal or serosubmucosal technique; all layers are included with the exception of the mucosa. A seromuscular stitch apposing and sealing the serous layers was described in 1826 by the Parisian surgeon Antoine Lembert (1802–1851), to prevent leakage; it does not incorporate the submucosa and is usually considered suitable only as a second-layer stitch.

Fig. 4.51 If the ends are disparate in calibre, cut back the narrower end on the side opposite the mesentery or the entry of the blood supply.

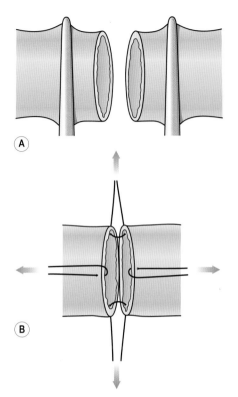

Fig. 4.52 Preparing to form an anastomosis. **A** Non-crushing bowel clamps steady the ends and prevent leakage of content. Some clamps can be locked together. **B** The ends are held together with traction sutures. If the bowel cannot be rotated, insert these not at the ends but slightly onto the back wall, so that when they are distracted they tauten the apposed back walls, leaving the anterior walls slack so that the back wall stitches can be easily inserted. (I was taught this method by Mr John Cochrane.) You may distract the anterior walls with stitches or tissue forceps to improve access to the posterior walls.

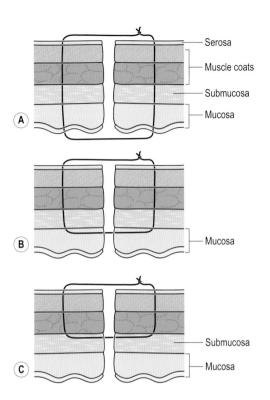

Fig. 4.53 A The all-coats stitch. **B** An extramucosal or serosubmucosal stitch. **C** The seromuscular or Lembert stitch. The knots are offset from the joined bowel edges.

4. Use a synthetic absorbable 3/0 suture mounted on a curved, round-bodied eyeless needle. Smooth monofilament material, having no interstices where organisms can reside, is safer in the presence of contamination but is a little stiff to tie. Braided multifilament suture is supple and forms reliable knots.

5. The method of stitching depends on personal choice and on the need to control the apposition of the edges. Use continuous, interrupted simple or mattress stitches passed vertically through all coats, 3–4 mm from the edge, 3–4 mm apart. Full-thickness interrupted and spiral continuous stitches are more haemostatic than mattress stitches. In either case carefully pick up and ligate bleeding vessels before starting the anastomotic suture.

6. The anastomotic line may lie in the sagittal or coronal planes. If the line of sutures lies in the sagittal plane it is usually easier to work from far to near; if it lies in the coronal plane it is usually easier to start at the end from your non-dominant to your dominant side.

7. It is also usually easier to drive the needle progressively from far to near when it lies in the transverse plane, from dominant to non-dominant side when it lies in the sagittal plane. In each case your hand starts fully pronated and drives the curved needle through by progressively supinating.

8. Your intention must be to appose the edges perfectly, just bringing into contact the same layers of each edge. The stitches cause inflammation, producing oedema. If you have pulled the stitches too tight, they cut off the blood supply and result in delayed healing, ulceration of the mucosa, or worse, cutting out with potential leakage.

9. The methods I shall describe are applicable throughout the bowel, but be prepared to practise the methods of your trainers.

10. On completion, check that the lumen is patent; carefully confirm that you can invaginate the walls from each side through the anastomotic ring.

Key points

- Check the colour of the bowel, the integrity of the blood supply, the lack of tension, the luminal continuity and the circumferential perfection of the union.
- If there is a mesentery to be closed, exclude haematoma that may subsequently prejudice healing.

11. Repair any defect in the mesentery with fine, interrupted sutures carefully inserted to avoid pricking any of the vessels or including them in the sutures and thus obliterating them.

Alternative methods

Used depending on the circumstances and on individual choice.

Mobile bowel, edge to edge, single layer, interrupted stitches

1. Insert sutures joining the anterior walls. Carefully avoid picking up the back wall. Tie the knots on the outside of the bowel.
2. When you have completed the anterior wall, turn the bowel over, to bring what was the back wall to the front and insert a series of sutures to close this, completing the anastomosis (Fig. 4.54).
3. If you used stay sutures, cut these out or tie them.
4. Carefully check the mesenteric and antimesenteric edges of the bowel – the junctions of the anterior and posterior suture lines are most likely to have defects. Insert extra sutures if necessary.

Edge to edge, single layer, continuous stitches

1. Starting on the back wall, insert a stitch at one end from outside in on one side, inside out on the other side and tie it. Clip the short end, insert the needle back through into the lumen and introduce a

continuous, unlocked, spiral stitch joining the back walls as far as the other end.

2. If the line of anastomosis lies in the sagittal plane, start at the near end, complete the stitching of the back wall, continue round the far corner and close the anterior walls from far to near, to reach the starting point. If you continue the spiral stitch onto the anterior wall you will discover you have to stitch with an unnatural action, starting with your hand held supine and pronating it to drive the stitch through. For a right-handed surgeon, to avoid this, at the far end, having passed the needle through to the left side, reverse the needle and pass it from within out, creating a loop on the mucosa – a single 'Connell' stitch. You can now continue to sew naturally, driving the needle from right to left along the anterior wall, to reach the starting point. Remove and discard the needle and tie the free end to the clamped short end. Reverse this if you are left-handed.

Fig. 4.55 Bowel anastomosis by continuous suture. The anastomotic line lies transversely. Start at the right side, insert an all-coats stitch and tie it. Enter the needle from without in on the near side. Unite the back walls with a spiral over-and-over stitch. At the left end insert a single Connell stitch on the near side and then continue from left to right on the anterior wall, to reach the first stitch and tie off. If you rotate the drawing 90° to the right (clockwise) it demonstrates the method when the anastomotic line lies in the sagittal plane.

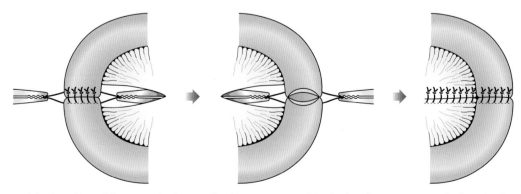

Fig. 4.54 If the bowel is mobile, suture the front wall, taking care to avoid the back wall. Now turn over the bowel to bring the previous back wall to the front and close it. If the bowel has a mesentery, carefully close the defect.

3. If the line of anastomosis lies in the transverse (coronal) plane, start at the right end (Fig. 4.55). Insert the first stitch from without in, then from within out, tie the stitch and clamp the short end. Reinsert the needle from without in on the near side. Carry on with the over and over spiral stitches, uniting the back walls from right to left. Again, at the left end, having taken the last stitch from far to near, reverse the needle to create a single Connell (mattress stitch with a loop on the mucosal aspect) stitch, coming out on the near side. You can now continue on the anterior suture line from left to right, inserting stitches from far to near. When you reach the right end, cut off the needle and tie the free end to the clamped short end.

4. Check that the anastomosis is patent.

Fixed bowel, single layer, interrupted stitches

1. This method is particularly applicable in the large bowel to anastomose it with the rectum, which lies against the sacrum and cannot be rotated. In addition, access is limited, so you must fashion the anastomosis not at the surface but in the depths.

> ### Key points
>
> - Do not unite the bowel ends under tension or they will surely distract.
> - Take particular care when inserting and tying sutures in situations that are inaccessible following completion of the procedure. This applies particularly to the posterior layer sutures in colorectal anastomoses.

2. Unite the posterior layers using carefully placed all-coats stitches, with the knots tied within the lumen. If the bowel is fixed, and subsequent access will be greatly restricted, place and tie these stitches with the bowel ends apart, clipping but not tying them until they are all inserted. Now, keeping the sutures taut and in the correct order, slide the mobile end down to lie accurately apposed to the fixed edge of bowel and tie them (Fig. 4.56). This is the 'parachute' technique. Leave the outer ligature ends long for the present but cut the ligature ends of the remainder, leaving the knots on the interior of the bowel.

3. Many colorectal surgeons use inverting, longitudinal (vertical) mattress sutures for the back wall (see Ch. 3). These pass out through all coats at a distance from the edge, enter the other bowel end at a similar distance from the edge, then take a small bite of each of the edges before being tied within the lumen.

4. Insert interrupted inverting anterior stitches to complete the anastomosis. These may be simple or inverting longitudinal mattress stitches. Because I was taught that bowel must be sutured using all-coats stitches as a basis I should favour these. Many colorectal surgeons employ extramucosal or even seromuscular stitches with success.

5. There are no absolute tests of perfection of the colorectal anastomosis but since it transmits solid faeces, many surgeons try to exclude defects or leaks that might disrupt the union or allow leakage with consequent infection. A reliable assistant may insert a finger through the anus to feel the integrity of the anastomosis and insert a narrow bore rigid sigmoidoscope and inspect it. Finally, the pelvis may

Fig. 4.56 If the bowel cannot be rotated, insert the back wall stitches, tying the knots within the lumen. In case of difficulty, leave the ends apart while you insert all the back wall stitches, slide the mobile end along the stitches and only then tie the knots. This is the 'parachute' technique.

anas

be filled with sterile saline and the rectal stump is gently inflated with air through the sigmoidoscope. If no bubbles appear, this suggests the anastomosis is satisfactory.

Two-layer anastomosis

In the past the stomach and bowel were routinely and very satisfactorily sutured using two layers. The inner, all-coats stitch inverts the bowel wall. This is reinforced with an absorbable or non-absorbable outer seromuscular Lembert stitch. Although most surgeons have converted to single-layer techniques, many senior surgeons, adept in the two-layer technique, continue to use it and obtain good results with it.

Variations

1. Anastomoses can be made not only end-to-end but also end-to-side and side-to-side (Fig. 4.57). In each circumstance ensure that the holes match each other.
2. Mechanical stapling devices are frequently used for joining bowel. Some, like the circular stapler, invert the bowel and apply a double row of metal staples. Others, like some straight stapling devices, apply a double row of staples to the everted edges; if necessary the staple line may be oversewn. When stitching is difficult to perform, mechanical methods are often more convenient. Do not assume, though, that mechanical devices can always be used more rapidly or more effectively than hand sewing. They demand careful placement.

Fig. 4.57 In addition to end-to-end anastomoses, the bowel can be joined end-to-side and side-to-side.

Key points

- Successful surgeons who employ techniques that work well for them often attribute their success to the method, but other successful surgeons using different techniques also pay tribute to their method.
- What is the explanation?
- The surgeons are too modest. Their success depends more on their skilful application of different but sound methods than on the techniques themselves.

Other ducts

1. Ureters undergo peristalsis to transmit the content. This may be impaired if the myenteric nerves or vascular supply are damaged. It is often worth cutting the ends obliquely to obviate producing an annular, constricting anastomosis.
2. Bile ducts have insufficient muscle in their walls to constrict, so they transmit contents passively by *vis a tergo* (force from behind). If they are injured, they often require to be united to another conduit, such as the jejunum. Bile is extremely penetrating and leaks if the anastomosis is imperfect.
3. Anastomosis of the fallopian tubes and vas deferens in order to restore continuity following disease or previous division is usually carried out using magnification.
4. Anastomosis of small ducts is almost always performed using a single row of interrupted, all-coats sutures. The fear is that a continuous encircling suture may have a constricting effect.

Key point

- Every stitch must unite the epithelial linings of the anastomosis. Fail, and a leak or stricture will follow.

5. Use a fine needle and suture to produce perfect, leak-free union. A straightforward end-to-end union produces a potential annular constriction ring. The postoperative oedema may block the lumen and rising pressure can then rupture the anastomosis with subsequent leakage. To avoid this, the anastomosis can be made over a 'T-tube' or straight tube (Fig. 4.58). If necessary, check the anastomosis and the 'run off', using radio-opaque contrast medium before you withdraw a splinting tube. The leakage from the side hole will rapidly heal provided there is no distal obstruction. A double pigtailed catheter can conveniently be inserted into a repaired ureter with the upper loop in the pelvis of the ureter and the lower one in the bladder (Fig. 4.13); it can be captured and extracted using a cystoscope.

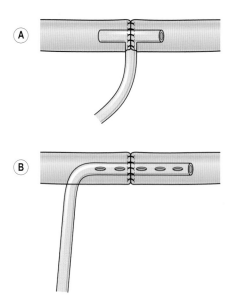

Fig. 4.58 **A** Insert a T-tube at the site of the anastomosis to splint the union. This channels the contents through the anastomosis or drains it externally. **B** The same effect is achieved by inserting a straight tube with side holes.

Fig. 4.60 Slit the end of a small duct to produce a wide opening. **A** Join it to another small duct, similarly split. **B** Join it to the end of a wide duct. **C** Join it into the side of a wide duct.

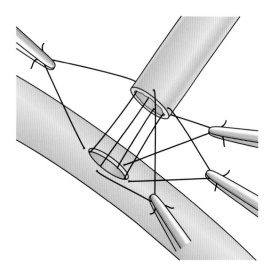

Fig. 4.59 Epithelium-to-epithelium anastomosis of small ducts is achieved by inserting the stitches while the ducts lie apart, then sliding one duct down onto the other.

6. If access is difficult as in the depths, place the stitches while the ducts lie apart before sliding them together – the 'parachute' technique (Fig. 4.59).
7. Be willing to slit the end of a small duct so that you can join it into a similar duct that has also been slit. The slit duct can also be joined to the end or side of a wide duct (Fig. 4.60). If necessary use stay sutures to hold the ducts in apposition while you insert the stitches.

8. You may close the end of a large open-ended duct until it will fit the end of a small duct. Alternatively, close the end completely, joining the small duct into a freshly made side opening (Fig. 4.61). Very small ducts are best cannulated with a plastic catheter which is tied in, before using the catheter as an introducer. If you leave the needled suture intact following ligation, pass the needle into the accepting hole and out nearby, so you can tie the end to the other end of the ligature to fix the duct in place. To prevent leakage, insert a purse-string suture around the anastomosis, gently push in the duct and tie the purse-string suture, producing an 'inkwell' effect.

BOWEL TRANSFER

Bowel, which has a rich blood supply, can be transferred to a different site but must retain or regain a blood supply to survive. A segment of bowel can be transferred elsewhere, while preserving its blood supply, by opening out the arching blood vessels that run in its mesentery to supply it from one end. The other end can be extended (Fig. 4.62). This was first described by the brilliant Swiss surgeon César Roux (1851–1934) in 1908. If it is necessary to transfer the segment at a distance, the blood vessels can be divided and reimplanted into vessels near the recipient site (Fig. 4.63). This demands highly skilled microvascular surgery (see Ch. 5).

Fig. 4.61 Joining small ducts into larger ones. **A** End-to-end. **B** End-to-side. **C** Using a plastic cannula to aid union of a small duct with a large one.

SPHINCTERS

Localized segments of specially controlled circular muscle meter and regulate the rate and direction of flow. These are sphincters (G *sphingein* = to bind tightly). They may or may not be anatomically obvious.

Inadvertent damage to the muscle or nerve supply may be irrevocable. Dilatation or overstretching often puts the sphincter out of action. It can be achieved in a similar manner to correcting a stricture, by passing graded bougies or balloon dilatation. The method may be used for achalasia (G *a* – not + *chalaein* = to relax) of the gastro-oesophageal cardia and to temporarily overcome anal sphincter spasm from anal fissure. If the sphincter is overstretched the muscle is disrupted and may never recover. If the muscle is torn the resulting fibrosis may produce stenosis.

Myotomy

1. Divide a clearly defined circular muscle forming a sphincter, using a longitudinal incision while leaving the lining intact (Fig. 4.64). Perform this when the sphincter is overdeveloped, or fails to relax, so that the contents cannot pass.

Fig. 4.62 Transferring bowel while retaining its blood supply. At the top on the left, the dotted lines show the lines of section, retaining the arterial circuit; on the right is a gap in the bowel to be bridged. At the bottom, the loop has been straightened out and joined in to bridge the gap on the right. The cut ends of the supplying bowel have been united to restore continuity on the left, with closure of the mesenteric defect.

Fig. 4.63 Bowel removed from one site has its blood vessels joined into those at the new site. As a rule, two veins are anastomosed for each artery.

2. *Infantile hypertrophic pyloric stenosis* can be treated by pyloromyotomy, described by Karl Ramstedt of Munster in 1912, which may be performed under local or general anaesthesia. Gently lift out

77

Fig. 4.64 Myotomy. Divide the sphincter (**A**) along the dotted line. Split the edges apart (**B**) to ensure that the circular muscle is totally divided. Leave the mucosal lining intact.

Fig. 4.65 Sphincterotomy. **A** Introduce one blade of the scissors into the mouth of the duct to cut through the encircling sphincter. **B** Introduce a grooved probe into the duct and cut down onto it with a scalpel.

the pylorus with fingers or tissue forceps. Hold it steady while carefully incising the thickened muscle, leaving the mucosa intact and bulging into the gap. Gently elevate remaining fibres using a hook or fine non-toothed forceps and cut them. Pick up each side of the cut edge using gauze swabs to improve your grip and gently separate the edges, or use round-nosed forceps to lever the edges apart. Sometimes you can collect a little air into the segment to bulge the mucosa and exclude or identify any leak. If there is a break in the mucosa, carefully suture it, perhaps drawing over it a tag of tissue such as omentum.

3. Myotomy of the lower oesophageal sphincter overcomes the condition of achalasia of the cardia of the stomach. Like pyloromyotomy, it is intended that the underlying mucosa remains intact. The operation was described by Ernst Heller of Leipzig in 1913.

Sphincterotomy

1. Divide the whole thickness, including the duct lining, when the sphincter controls the termination of a spouted duct (Fig. 4.65). The ampulla of Abraham Vater (1684–1751 of Wittemberg in Germany) usually accepts both the common bile and pancreatic ducts. Through an opening in the duodenum, insinuate one blade of a pair of scissors into the spout and cut through with the other blade. Alternatively, pass in a grooved probe and cut down into the groove with a scalpel. This type of sphincterotomy is now usually performed through a fibreoptic endoscope, using a diathermy wire.

2. *Fistula in ano* is usually between the rectum or anus and the skin of the perineum and may require sphincterotomy to treat it (see below).

3. *Anal fissure* can sometimes be successfully treated by the application of local anaesthetic combined with stool-softening agents, application of glyceryl trinitrate (GTN) or injection of type A botulinum toxin (Botox) 20 units diluted to 50 units/mL. If these fail it can usually be successfully treated by dividing the lower internal sphincter. The fissure nearly always lies in the midline posteriorly but carry out the sphincterotomy on the lateral wall. Insert a proctoscope with an open slot that reveals the lateral anal wall. Make a small circumferential incision at the anal margin. Through this insert closed blunt-ended scissors beneath the mucosa and gently open them to separate the mucosa and lower internal sphincter. Withdraw the scissors, close them and again insert them, this time deep to the lower internal sphincter, and open them to separate it from the external sphincter. Remove the scissors and introduce a straight haemostat, one blade superficial to, one blade deep to the internal sphincter, clamp it, open it and withdraw it. With the scissors now cut vertically through the crushed sphincter to the upper level of the fissure.

4. *Episiotomy* (G *epision* = pubic region + *tome* = a cutting). There is no closure sphincter at the lower end of the vagina but during parturition (L *parare* = to bring forth), the skin and circular muscle of the lower vagina may be torn, with a risk of uncontrollable extension. To avoid this the obstetrician (L *ob* = before + *stare* = to stand) may deliberately cut the tissues to divert any tear clear of the anus, carefully repairing it after the baby is delivered.

Sphincteroplasty

If you perform sphincterotomy, the raw edges may rejoin. However, if you join the inner and outer epithelia with sutures, the opening will remain patulous (Fig. 4.66). When a sphincter surrounds a duct in continuity, such as the pylorus, incise longitudinally through it, widely separate the walls and suture the defect as a transverse suture line. At the pylorus this manoeuvre is referred to as a *pyloroplasty*. It is a method of overcoming stenosis that results from chronic peptic ulcer in the proximal duodenum with consequent scar contracture.

Sphincter repair

A sphincter may need to be cut deliberately. Repairs of old sphincteric defects or tears are usually less successful; it is occasionally effective to excise the edges of the old, scarred sphincter and carry out a fresh repair (Fig. 4.67).

Sphincter reversal

Some sphincters act unidirectionally, rather like valves. Indeed, as a rule, though not always, the direction of peristaltic action in the bowel is unidirectional so that it acts

Fig. 4.66 Sphincteroplasty. **A** Divide a terminal sphincter and stitch the inner and outer linings together. **B** Divide the sphincter longitudinally, widely separate the edges and sew up the defect as a transverse suture line.

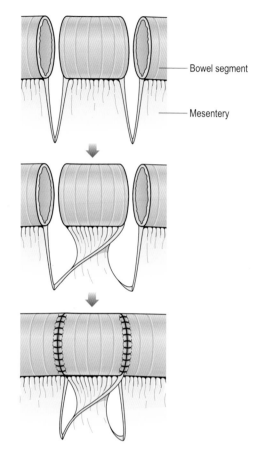

Fig. 4.67 Sphincter repair. Excise the edges to expose the fresh, raw ends of the sphincter before suturing them together.

Bowel segment

Mesentery

Fig. 4.68 Sphincter reversal. Take out of continuity the sphincteric segment, still attached to its blood supply, reverse it and restore it into continuity.

like a one-way valve. In order to slow down the passage in the hope of allowing more time for absorption following massive bowel resection, it is possible to take out a segment, still attached by its blood and nerve supply, reverse it, and restore it into continuity (Fig. 4.68).

ACQUIRED CHANNELS AND CAVITIES

These are varied in origin including developmental, traumatic, infective, resulting from the presence of foreign material, and neoplastic.

Sinus

(L = something hollowed out, a bay.)
1. The lining of the channel may be granulation tissue but it may become epithelialized. In some cases removing the cause may suffice, in others the whole track needs to be excised.

79

2. The most common sinus you will see is a *wound sinus*. A superficial stitch often acts as a foreign body, especially if it has a long, stiff cut end lying beneath the skin which eventually protrudes. In some cases it may be caused by a piece of necrotic tissue or missed foreign material. Initially try to insert sinus forceps or fine 'mosquito' artery forceps, gently open the blades and attempt to capture the stitch or other cause and remove it. If this fails, be willing to explore the sinus under local anaesthesia, enlarging the opening until you can see the cause and remove it.

3. A classical condition is *pilonidal sinus* (L *pilum* = hair + *nidus* = nest). Hair driven beneath the skin over the coccyx forms a source of chronic irritation and often infection. It has an external opening. In the past it was often widely excised as though it was a malignancy. It is now usually treated successfully by opening up the channel to the surface, scrupulously removing all the hairs, and keeping the mouth widely open while the cavity fills up from the depths (Fig. 4.69) to obliterate itself.

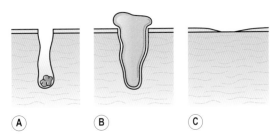

Fig. 4.69 Sinus. **A** A sinus with foreign material, diseased tissue, or hair within a pilonidal sinus. **B** The irritant cause of chronicity has been removed, the opening has been widened and the cavity packed so that it fills the base. **C** The base has filled with granulation tissue, which contracts while epithelium grows in to heal over.

Fistula

1. The term fistula (L = pipe) is used in medicine to signify a pipe open at both ends onto an epithelial surface. In some cases removing the cause may succeed but if the track becomes completely epithelialized it will never close spontaneously. When the lobe of an ear is pierced and an earring inserted, epithelium grows through, and lines the track, so that it will remain open for life. If there is infection, foreign material, neoplasia and a high rate of flow through the track it is unlikely to heal, especially if the discharge is irritant. This applies if a fistula develops from, for example, the biliary system or the bowel. The fistula will never heal if there is distal obstruction and the fistulous track is acting as a safety channel.

2. In some circumstances, as when a fistulous tract relieves an impassable or unresectable obstruction, the fistula is beneficial. If a serious leakage occurs into a large compartment such as the peritoneal cavity, containment as a result of the development of a fistulous track spares the patient possible generalized peritonitis.

3. A *fistula in ano* results from inflammation usually in or near the lower bowel, although it may develop from more proximal intestine. Infection may result in an abscess which sometimes 'points' towards the perianal skin so that a track develops between the bowel and skin. A probe can usually be passed from the external orifice, through the track into the bowel. If the track is now laid open (Fig. 4.70) and subsequently kept open until new tissue has filled the defect it may heal. This cannot always be achieved if the internal opening is high, because it entails dividing too much of the anal sphincter muscles that maintain anal continence.

   The standard method is to pass a probe through the track, usually from the perianal skin into the anus, then cut down onto the probe so that the whole length of the track is exposed. Such treatment transects

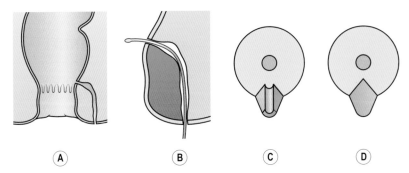

Fig. 4.70 Fistula. **A** Diagram of an anal fistulous track communicating between the anal canal and the perianal skin. **B** A malleable probe has been passed through the track and the intervening tissue has been divided (shaded portion), exposing the track in the bottom of the cleft you have created (**C**) when seen from the perineal aspect. **D** As a result of the packing and other measures to prevent the edges from bridging over, the cleft is shallow, smaller, and will shortly heal.

intervening sphincteric muscle. The operation demands skill and experience to avoid excessive damage to the sphincteric muscle layers, rendering the anus incompetent. In some cases extensive muscle division can be averted by first constricting the tissue to be divided within a ligature (a seton), which causes fibrosis so that when the muscle is transected the fibres are held by the scar tissue and do not retract.

Stoma

1. The term stoma (G = mouth) applies to a natural or artificial mouth between an internal duct and another duct, another part of the same channel, or to the exterior. For example, the mouth is a natural stoma, surgical union of the stomach and intestine is a gastroenterostomy (G *enteron* = L intestine from *intus* = within), the exteriorization of the colon to the skin is a colostomy.
2. Provided the lining of the two surfaces fuse, the stoma is stable. If fusion does not occur, or if the epithelium is destroyed, fibrosis develops and as this matures it contracts so that the stoma constricts. For this reason, if you wish to form a permanent stoma as when joining intestine at an anastomosis, joining ducts, or uniting a duct into the bowel, ensure that the epithelium and mucosa are sutured into perfect contact. When forming a colostomy (Fig. 4.71), mucosa and skin must be carefully united. In the past surgeons often brought bowel to the surface without uniting the mucosa to skin. As a result a frequently performed operation was 'refashioning of colostomy'.

Cysts

1. Some cysts (G *kystis* = bladder, bag or pouch) are developmental such as **branchial cyst** (G *branchion* = gill). If an epithelium such as skin is detached and buried, it grows until it meets other cells of the same tissue, resulting in an **implantation cyst**. Some diseases, including neoplasms, result in cyst formation.
2. One method of dealing with a cyst is to excise it without opening it, avoiding spilling the contents. This applies to **ovarian, branchial** and **epididymal** (G *epi* = upon + *didymos* = twin; it was an old term for both testes and ovaries) cysts. A retention cyst such as a sebaceous cyst can usually be excised under local anaesthesia; prefer to use a fairly large volume of dilute anaesthetic injected not into but around the cyst. This separates the capsule from the surrounding tissue, greatly facilitating the subsequent sharp dissection and reducing bleeding. If you fail to excise all the secretory lining of a cystic gland, it is liable to reform.
3. The most common cyst with which you will have to deal is a **sebaceous cyst** (L *sebum* = fat, suet; see Ch. 6).
4. A retention cyst near a surface can often be decapitated by removing the overlying tissue. The epithelium of the surface rapidly fuses with the lining of the cyst (Fig. 4.72). Salivary cysts within the mouth are amenable to this treatment.
5. Occasionally a cavity such as a cyst can be treated by introducing a tube attached to a suction device which draws the walls together so that it collapses and shrivels.

Abscesses

See Chapter 12.

Fig. 4.71 External stoma. Diagram through a stoma in which the end of the bowel has been brought to the surface through a hole made in the abdominal wall. The end of the bowel wall has been everted so that the mucosa can be stitched directly to the skin.

(A) (B) (C)

Fig. 4.72 De-roofing a cyst. **A** A retention cyst: the secretions cannot escape because the mouth of the glandular cyst is stenosed. **B** The overlying epithelium and the roof of the cyst have been removed. **C** The lining of the cyst and the epithelium have fused at the edges and the surface gradually becomes uniform.

Chapter | 5 |

Handling blood vessels

1. The anatomical arrangement of the main blood vessels provides general protection from injury and overstretching. Those in the trunk lie posteriorly close to the vertebrae, cushioned anteriorly by the viscera. In the limbs they lie on the flexor surfaces of joints.

2. Transmission of blood is by *vis a tergo* (L *vis* = force, compulsion + *tergum* = the back; hence, compulsion from behind). Blood vessels do not undergo peristalsis. Blood flow is not uniform within the lumen. The central, axial stream, carrying the cells and larger molecules, is faster than the peripheral blood which is subject to the 'drag' of the intima. The smooth flow of blood may be disturbed by turbulence, especially if there is irregularity of the intimal lining. The size of the channel does not automatically respond to the volume of fluid passing through it – arteries or veins may constrict as a result of autonomic-system-driven smooth muscle contraction, at a time when there is an increased demand for vascular transport.

3. The internal surface of blood vessels is lined with endothelial cells forming a continuous surface. If these intimal cells are damaged, destroyed or separated by over-distension to expose the subintimal collagen, platelets adhere and trigger clotting factors. In the presence of local inflammation the intimal cells express the cell adhesion molecule E-selectin, which binds to certain leukocytes and causes them to adhere to and pass through the endothelium to reach the site of inflammation.

4. Arteries (G *arteria* = windpipe – after death the arteries are empty and were thought to transmit air) have a substantial medial layer of smooth muscle

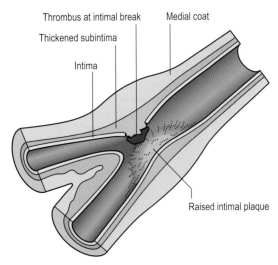

Fig. 5.1 Atheroma at site of arterial division producing turbulence. Macrophages containing low-density lipoproteins accumulate in the subintima. The medial smooth muscle layer thickens and may dilate. At breaks in the intimal plaques, platelets and thrombus adhere to the subintimal layer.

Labels on figure: Thrombus at intimal break; Medial coat; Thickened subintima; Intima; Raised intimal plaque

cells. In susceptible patients macrophages containing low-density lipoprotein (LDL) are deposited beneath the intima in arteries, especially at sites of turbulence such as bifurcations. Veins are affected only when they are substituted as arterial grafts, bypasses and at arteriovenous fistulas. The deposition produces atheromatous (G *athara* = porridge + -*oma* = tumour or swelling) plaques which may calcify and which raise the intima, encroaching on the lumen (Fig. 5.1). In addition, the medial coat of smooth muscle thickens and may expand and eventually become aneurysmal (G *ana* = up + *eurys* = wide). If the intimal cells are swept off the plaques, platelets adhere and expose the vessel to thrombus formation and possible stenosis or obstruction. If blood undermines the exposed intimal edge, a flap may be progressively raised that results in blood flow in a true and false lumen – a dissection. The texture of the vessel becomes irregular, friable and difficult to suture securely.

5. Vein walls have a thin smooth muscle media, since the pressure within them is normally low. Many are valved so that they transmit blood in only one direction. Because the blood flow is usually slower than in arteries, there is an increased tendency for clotting to occur if the endothelium is damaged, if there is stagnation, or if there is a clotting diathesis (G *diatithenai* = to dispose – a predisposition). Obstruction to venous return causes distension. During pregnancy, intrapelvic pressure from the enlarged uterus compresses pelvic veins, dilating lower limb veins, widening the valve rings, so the valves become incompetent, creating varicose veins; the congestion may also distend the haemorrhoidal veins. Hepatic portal venous obstruction distends the portal-systemic anastomoses especially at the gastro-oesophageal junction.

6. During, and following surgical operations on the blood vessels, clots are likely to form because of trauma, minute breaks in intimal continuity, stagnation, the presence of sutures and clotting diathesis.

7. Local anticoagulation reduces the likelihood, especially in arterial surgery, using 500 mL isotonic saline containing 5000 international units (IU) heparin to flush and instil topically.

PERCUTANEOUS PUNCTURE

Veins

Key points

- Your skill in gaining access to veins is frequently called on, often in emergency circumstances with collapsed deeply placed veins. Practise, practise, practise.
- Do not attempt venepuncture until you have confidently identified the anatomy or you put at risk adjacent arteries, nerves and other vital structures. Learn and use every aid.
- Repeated failure erodes your confidence and that of your patient. Seek help.

1. Veins are most easily cannulated when they are distended. They constrict in hypovolaemia, exposure to cold, and as a result of local trauma. Veins distend if they are warm, if they are placed dependently, or mildly congested; this can often be achieved by simple finger pressure restricting venous return. In the limbs, place a cuff that obstructs venous return but not arterial inflow, and the effect can be augmented if the subject performs repeated muscle contractions of the part. Use a warm hot water bottle or hair dryer to encourage local venous filling.

2. Do not over-congest veins, especially in elderly people; they rupture spontaneously or when punctured.

3. Ensure that the lighting is adequate – tangential lighting may be helpful by producing shadowing of the dilated vein. Be prepared to shave overlying hair to improve the view. A deeply sited vein can often be identified if you place one finger over the likely site. Gently tap proximally or peripherally, or for some sites ask the patient to cough. Your 'watching' finger detects the thrill. Some veins can be identified because descriptions exist of their anatomical

position, with recommendations of site, direction and depth of needle insertion. Internal jugular, subclavian and femoral vein punctures are examples; the saphenous vein is reliably found 3.5 cm (1½") directly above the tip of the tibial medial malleolus, although this is not a favoured site for venepuncture. It is now recommended that for central line insertion, a Doppler ultrasound probe is used to aid insertion.

4. If you must insert a large needle, or carry out a subsequent manoeuvre, and especially if the patient is apprehensive, do not hesitate to inject a small volume of local anaesthetic intracutaneously through a fine needle; a 29 gauge needle attached to an insulin syringe has been suggested. Form at first a superficial bleb at a spot you can identify when the fluid has been absorbed. Allow a few minutes for it to take effect, then insert the needle through the site of the bleb. Before inserting a large needle or one carrying an external cannula, first make a small incision with a pointed scalpel. The needle then slides easily through the superficial tissues and the 'feel' is not lost, as it is when the needle is tightly gripped by skin (Fig. 5.2). Apply a finger or thumb just beside the vein and draw it distally, slightly stretching the vessel to keep it in line.

5. Elderly patients often may present two difficulties. As some veins are distended and then punctured, they rupture and bleed into the tissues, obstructing the view. Avoid over-distending them. Others are thick-walled, slippery, and difficult to fix while puncturing them. Look for a junction which tethers the vein (Fig. 5.3).

6. If you press too close to the vein or apply too strong traction, you will collapse it and your finger obstructs the line of needle insertion. When the site of insertion lies near a joint, exert gentle traction by bending the joint (Fig. 5.4).

Fig. 5.3 The needle is about to enter a superficial vein at the junction of tributaries, where the draining vessel is relatively fixed. The right hand holding the syringe is omitted.

Cephalic vein — — Basilic vein

Bicipital aponeurosis

Fig. 5.2 The medial basilic vein, separated from the brachial artery by the bicipital aponeurosis, is a popular site for venepuncture. The proximal quick release tourniquet congests the veins, your left thumb to one side of the vein steadies it without compressing it. The right hand is omitted. Hold the syringe and needle almost flat with the skin, needle bevel uppermost.

Fig. 5.4 If the vein lies near a joint you can flex it. This slightly stretches and fixes the vein, offering you a clear view along it.

7. Insert the needle, with the bevel uppermost, almost vertically through the skin, since the longer its track within the skin, the more uncomfortable the prick. Now direct it so that it lies close to, and parallel to, the vein. Angle the tip so that it 'squashes' gently into the vein to enter the lumen (Fig. 5.5). Check this by gently aspirating blood into the syringe, then advance the needle within the vein but avoid introducing the whole needle; if it breaks at the Luer connection the shaft cannot be grasped and withdrawn.

> **Key point**
>
> - Do not withdraw the needle until you have removed the congesting cuff.

8. Apply gentle pressure through a sterile swab over the puncture site while you extract the needle and maintain the pressure for 3 minutes, timed by the clock.
9. Do not rely on needles for long-term infusion into veins. Needles soon pull out, or penetrate the vein wall allowing the fluid to 'tissue'.
10. When you require repeated access, as for haemodialysis in patients with chronic renal failure, you will need to create an arteriovenous fistula, anastomosing the radial or brachial artery to the cephalic vein. The increased pressure in the vein distends it so that it can be repeatedly cannulated.

Arteries

1. Arteries are often mobile and if they are thick walled in elderly or hypertensive people they may slip from under a needle or be difficult to puncture.
2. Raise a bleb of local anaesthetic in the skin at the site of puncture and infiltrate the tissues around the artery. Make a small stab through the skin with a pointed scalpel blade. This important step allows you to slide the needle easily down to the vessel, so that you can 'feel' the entry into it; only now is it gripped as you advance it.
3. Fix the artery if possible by pressing it against a firm base (Fig. 5.6).
4. Insert the needle with the bevel uppermost until it lies on the artery, then enter the artery at an angle, when small spurts of blood enter the syringe. The pressure required to puncture a thick-walled artery may collapse it, so make short jerky movements.
5. In case of difficulty it may be less damaging to transfix the artery cleanly and then slowly withdraw the needle until blood spurts into the syringe, rather than repeatedly stabbing into the thick wall (Fig. 5.7).
6. Needles are not suitable for prolonged retention in an artery since they damage the endothelium and may penetrate the vessel wall or become dislodged, allowing leakage to occur.
7. When you withdraw the needle have a sterile pad available to press on the puncture site; maintain this for at least 5 minutes timed by the clock, depending on the patient's clotting status.

Fig. 5.5 A Pierce the skin almost vertically. **B** Align the needle almost parallel to the vein and prepare to 'squash' it into the vein. Notice the bevel is uppermost. **C** View from above shows the needle in the line of the vein, exactly over it. **D** The needle enters the vein, accurately lined up with it.

Fig. 5.6 Percutaneous puncture of an artery. Locate and fix it with your non-dominant hand.

Fig. 5.7 Percutaneous arterial puncture. Rather than make repeated damaging attempts (**A**), transfix the artery, gradually withdraw the needle (**B**) until blood spurts into the syringe, then (**C**) advance the needle within the lumen of the artery.

Fig. 5.8 **A** The closely fitting cannula is smoothly chamfered distally onto the needle. **B** The needle enters the vessel; then hold it steady. **C** Advance the cannula over the needle. **D** Withdraw the needle, leaving the cannula in place.

PERCUTANEOUS CANNULATION

Cannula (L = reed) suggests a stiff tube. Most modern vascular cannulas are commercially produced plastic sheaths fitted closely on needles, the distal part of the cannula being chamfered smoothly onto the shank of the needle (Fig. 5.8). A disadvantage of this cannula is that it cannot be longer than the needle. However, it has the advantage over a needle in that the plastic cannula is unlikely to damage or perforate the vessel wall from within. Moreover, if it is of sufficient calibre, it provides an adequate channel for the passage of a variety of catheters, guidewires and other instruments.

Key point

- Never reintroduce a partially or completely withdrawn needle into the cannula. The needle may penetrate the plastic cannula wall, detach it, and create a foreign body embolus.

Veins

1. To introduce the cannula, proceed as for percutaneous puncture. First raise a bleb of local anaesthetic, wait 5 minutes then create a small punctured incision to accommodate the needle and cannula. When you enter the vein, gently advance it against the increasing resistance as the tip of the cannula smoothly expands the hole to enter the lumen. Be careful to maintain the tip of the needle central within the vein, to avoid damaging or perforating the wall.
2. When you are confident that the cannula has entered the vein, hold the needle still while gently advancing the cannula. Now withdraw the needle after preparing to connect or control the cannula.
3. If you are in doubt about the correct siting of the cannula, connect a syringe and confirm that blood can be aspirated.

Arteries

Key point

- Do not start until you have confidently identified the artery.

1. Proceed initially as for percutaneous venous cannulation. When you enter the artery, gently advance the cannula against the increasing resistance as its tip smoothly expands the hole to enter the lumen.
2. Be careful to maintain the tip of the needle central within the artery, to avoid damaging or perforating the wall.
3. Watch carefully for incipient leakage producing a haematoma, while you are trying to insert the needle and cannula. Withdraw the cannula and compress the site for 5 minutes by the clock. Move to a fresh site.

4. When you are confident that the cannula has entered the artery, gently advance it while holding the needle still. Now withdraw the needle after preparing to connect or control the cannula.
5. Confirm that blood spurts into the syringe.
6. Carefully and gently compress the entry site for 5 minutes timed by the clock.

PERCUTANEOUS CATHETERIZATION

Hippocrates used the term catheter (G *kata* = down + *hienai* = to send) for an instrument for emptying the bladder. Like cannulas, they were also stiff tubes until the French surgeon Auguste Nélaton invented the rubber catheter in 1860. Intravenous catheters are made of plastic tubing. They may be inserted into veins or arteries. They can be passed through needles or cannulas, provided their external diameter is less than the internal diameter of the needle or cannula (Fig. 5.9). When the needle is withdrawn it cannot be removed from the catheter if this has an external Luer connection unless the needle is of a special type that can be split longitudinally and opened.

Whereas cannulas that fit on the outside of needles are usually limited in length, catheters that can be introduced through a large-bore needle or cannula can be of unlimited length, so they can be introduced at a convenient site and passed for long distances to the required site.

Seldinger technique

1. The Swedish radiologist Sven-Ivar Seldinger (1921–1998) devised in 1953 a technique for percutaneous introduction of a catheter. Originally developed for arteries he extended it and it is now also valuable in almost every system for entering blood vessels, ducts, hollow viscera, natural or pathological spaces.

Fig. 5.9 Inserting a blunt catheter percutaneously using a sharp needle as a pilot. **A** A catheter passed through the lumen of the needle. **B** The needle withdrawn.

2. Initially inject local anaesthetic at the introduction site and make a small incision through which you will pass the needle, guidewire, and the catheter.
3. Introduce a hollow needle percutaneously into the vessel. If the internal calibre of the needle is insufficient, select one that carries an external, close-fitting, plastic cannula and withdraw the needle, leaving the cannula within the vessel (Fig. 5.10).
4. Through the needle or cannula pass a flexible, floppy-ended, round-tipped, guidewire into the lumen. Withdraw the needle or cannula, leaving the guidewire.
5. Pass over the guidewire a close-fitting but easy sliding catheter with a chamfered tip that will pass through the wall of the vessel.
6. If you need to pass a wide-bore catheter, first pass a series of graded plastic dilators so the largest one can carry the selected catheter (Fig. 5.11).
7. Advance the guidewire and catheter, usually under imaging control, to the target site.
8. A simple development of the technique has greatly increased the versatility and guidance of the catheter. If a catheter has a bend incorporated into the tip, the degree of bending can be reduced by inserting a straight guidewire. As the guidewire enters the curved portion, this is straightened (Fig. 5.12). The straightened catheter can be advanced, rotated and then allowed to regain curvature in order to enter, for example, a side channel. A range of preformed

Fig. 5.10 Seldinger's guidewire technique. **A** Cannulate the vessel. **B** Withdraw the needle and replace it with the guidewire. **C** Withdraw the cannula and replace it with the plastic catheter. **D** Remove the guidewire.

Fig. 5.12 A The straight guidewire alongside (**B**) the preformed curve-tipped catheter. **C** A catheter with a guidewire inserted through the straight portion of the catheter. **D** The straight guidewire is pushed into the preformed curved portion of the catheter, partially straightening it.

Fig. 5.11 A The Seldinger wire has been passed into the vessel. **B** Pass the dilator, carrying the insertion cannula, into the vessel, over the guidewire. **C** Withdraw the guidewire and dilator, leaving the cannula in place. **D** Pass the catheter through the cannula into the vessel. **E** Withdraw the cannula.

catheter shapes and shaped guidewires are available for passage through stenoses, occlusions, often at awkward angles – for example the superior mesenteric, renal and intracerebral arteries.

9. Catheters can be inserted for long distances and guided to specific points. Locate the tip by aspirating and identifying the contents of the lumen. If the catheter tip is radio-opaque it may be visible on plain X-rays, or an imaging medium may be injected through it and identified on X-rays.

10. The technique has opened up a large number of possible minimally invasive investigations and therapeutic procedures within the circulatory and other systems. An expert interventional radiologist can collect specimens, deliver substances, obtain pressure measurements and make a radiological or imaging diagnosis often with the aid of injected contrast medium. In addition, vessels can be selectively embolized, ablated and controlled (see below).

> **Key points**
>
> - Never lose control of the guidewire. If you do it may be swept into the vessel and become irrecoverable.
> - The guidewire maintains your access channel. Do not remove it until the procedure is complete.
> - Recognize the value of acquiring skill in manipulating the Seldinger wire and catheters. It is a classical illustration of a versatile technique applicable in a wide range of uses. Skills are transferable.

ENDOVASCULAR SURGERY

1. Approximately 70% of arterial conditions can now be treated by endoluminal methods.
2. The balloon-tipped catheter devised by Thomas Fogarty in the early 1960s can be introduced proximally into a blood vessel, and passed distally through and beyond a soft clot or embolus. The balloon is inflated and then when the catheter is gently withdrawn it brings the clot with it. If necessary it can be introduced over a guidewire. For adherent clot, especially in prosthetic vessels, Fogarty has introduced corkscrew-like clot-removing wires.

3. Selective angiography can be performed by negotiating the catheter tip to the specific site and injecting contrast medium for imaging. In the presence of bleeding as from, for example, subarachnoid haemorrhage or bleeding peptic ulcer, the bleeding vessel may be identified by angiography and platinum coils injected to occlude it.

4. Angioplasty balloons carried by catheters can be sited across stenoses and inflated to dilate the vessel. The catheters will distend to a predetermined diameter and rupture if over-inflated. Sizes extend from 1 to 2 mm diameter for distal lower limb vessel to occlusive balloons for the aorta. Narrowed carotid and coronary arteries can be dilated for the treatment of carotid artery stenosis and cardiac ischaemia, respectively.

5. After successful balloon angioplasty, endovascular stents may be inserted to maintain the channel, although reactive intimal hyperplasia may cause restenosis in up to one third of patients.

6. Endovascular aneurysm repair is performed using stent grafts made of polyester or polytetrafluoroethylene (PTFE) attached to a metal stent comprising either stainless steel or nickel titanium (nitinol). The grafts are introduced via the femoral arteries and deployed within the aneurysm. The metal stent provides radial and longitudinal support. The aneurysm is excluded from the circulation by the graft material.

7. Bleeding from gastro-oesophageal varices in portal venous hypertension resulting from hepatic cirrhosis can usually be controlled by transjugular intrahepatic portasystemic stent shunt (TIPSS). Under imaging control a catheter is passed over a guidewire through the right internal jugular vein, superior and inferior venae cavae to the right hepatic vein, through which a needle and then a guidewire connect it through the liver substance to the portal vein. A self-expanding metal stent is then placed across, creating a portal/systemic shunt. The procedure is usually performed under local anaesthesia.

SUTURES

1. Monofilament polyethylene or polyester-coated braided material are non-absorbable, as is polytetrafluoroethylene (PTFE), which is used when suturing grafts made of that material. Sutures are mounted on curved, round-bodied, taper-pointed, eyeless needles. For the aorta size 3/0 is used, with diminishing sizes as small as 8/0 for small arteries and veins. Sutures can be supplied with an attached needle at each end –'double needled'.

2. If the smooth surface of extruded, synthetic suture material is damaged, it is seriously weakened. Monofilament material is at greatest risk because

Fig. 5.13 Creation of a dissection. The arrow indicates the direction of blood flow.

a single break in the surface puts the whole thread at risk. Never grasp sutures with metal instruments except in segments that will be discarded, or drag them over hard, rough surfaces, or jerkily snatch them; you will reduce the strength by up to 50%. Extruded monofilament plastic threads have 'memory' and imperfectly locked knots tend to slip.

3. Insert sutures, whenever possible, from within out. Especially when suturing diseased arteries there is a danger that a needle passed from without in (Fig. 5.13) will separate the intima from the media. Blood can then insinuate itself beneath the endothelium, diverting the flow away from the lumen and causing progressive endothelial stripping – a 'dissection'. The danger is greatest when the intima is lifted on the peripheral side of a break in continuity in the direction of blood flow and therefore most likely to lift the endothelium. For this reason, when suturing a transverse defect in an artery, start from the outside in on the upstream side, and from the inside out on the downstream side.

4. Bear in mind when suturing diseased arteries that atheromatous plaques make the wall fragile. You may need to vary the regularity of the stitches to maintain both the integrity and haemostasis of the suture line.

5. Carefully follow the curve of the needle by rotating your needle-holder; if you do not you may tear out the needle or thread, or enlarge the hole, so creating a point of leakage.

6. Use non-toothed dissecting forceps held in your non-dominant hand to assist you when inserting sutures. Avoid gripping the vessel – and especially avoid grasping the endothelium. Use the forceps for counter pressure when inserting the needle; it is often convenient to allow the blades to separate slightly while you drive the needle through the vessel wall to emerge between them (Fig. 5.14).

7. Every stitch must pick up the endothelium and all layers. Every knot must be formed correctly and tightened correctly. The distance from the edges and between stitches depends on the size of the vessels.

8. Stitches may be:
    a. Continuous: unlocked stitches are the standard method of suturing. Since they form a spiral around the circumference of an artery,

Fig. 5.14 Use slightly open dissecting forceps for counter pressure as you drive the needle through the vessel wall, not as graspers.

each distending pulsation of the vessel tightens the spiral. Recovery of blood pressure following operation with arterial distension similarly tightens the spiral stitches, reducing the likelihood of leakage (Fig. 5.15A).

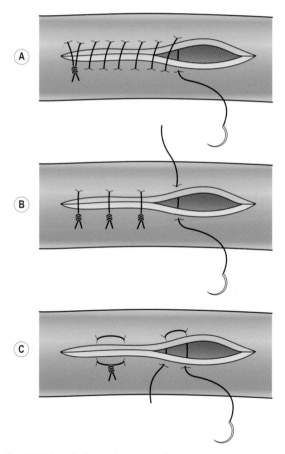

Fig. 5.15 A A single continuous spiral stitch. **B** Simple interrupted stitches, necessary when suturing very small calibre vessels. **C** An everting mattress stitch bringing together the endothelium from each side; it may be used to initiate eversion and can then often be continued using simple stitches.

b. Interrupted: single stitches are appropriate for small vessels and in paediatric surgery because they do not restrict increase in vessel circumference as growth proceeds (Fig. 5.15B). However, because stitch separation is increased when the vessel distends, there is an increased risk of bleeding if the stitches are not correctly placed, correctly tightened and tied.

c. Provided you can obtain perfect apposition of the intima, you should not evert the whole arterial wall with mattress stitches (Fig. 5.15C), which narrow the lumen (Fig. 5.16). Very occasionally it is valuable to start with a single mattress stitch to initiate eversion, or when suturing diseased arteries if a single stitch may cut out, or to start an anastomosis from the inside of the back wall of a fixed artery that cannot be rotated.

9. It is usually easier to insert sutures on a curved needle mounted in a needle-holder from far to near or from your dominant side to non-dominant side. You insert the needle with your hand fully pronated, progressively supinating it to drive the needle through to emerge near you, or to your non-dominant side. Follow the curve of the needle by a series of small 'pushes' through the tissue. If you merely drive it through, you will produce a large stitch hole, resulting in bleeding. Until you are skilled, be willing to move to the other side of the operating table in order to suture in a comfortable, practised manner.

10. The skill of inserting stitches and drawing them to the correct tension to seal the vessel cannot be transmitted indirectly – you must assiduously watch your masters and learn the correct tension – do not let them loosen. Pass the emerging thread to your assistant to hold without changing the tension.

Fig. 5.16 While it is essential for the intima to be picked up with every stitch so the edges on both sides meet, the whole vessel wall should not be everted or the lumen is reduced.

Repeated slackening and retightening of the thread exerts a sawing effect on the vessel wall, with a tendency to cut out. It also damages the thread surface, weakening it.

Key points

- You cannot acquire the necessary skill to suture blood vessels from this or any other book.
- You must assiduously watch, and practise under the eye of your masters.

11. Knots are invariably placed on the external surface. They are potential causes of failure if they are improperly tied, either because they are imperfectly formed or tightened, or there is an insufficient number of half-hitches, or because the material has been damaged by rough handling. The more knots, the more potential sites of failure. Tie as many as seven or eight correctly formed and fully tightened half-hitches, each successive one forming a reef knot with the previous one. Leave the ends long.

EXPOSE AND CONTROL (see also Ch. 10.)

1. Revise the anatomy beforehand, but remember that blood vessels do not always follow the usual path. Disease processes may distort and weaken vessels and surrounding tissue. Blood vessels and nerves frequently run together within a sheath. In exposing individual blood vessels avoid damaging other structures.
2. On many occasions veins are exposed for cosmetic reasons. Never fail to mark the intended site of incision beforehand. Place the incision to produce the best possible postoperative appearance compatible with safe exposure, preferably parallel to the skin tension lines.
3. When exposing veins to act as arterial bypass vessels, handle them as little as possible. It appears that leaving the cuff of adventitia intact with the vein, and manipulating the vein by grasping this rather than the vein itself, reduces the tendency to spasm.
4. Gently open round-nosed haemostatic forceps on each side to expose first one side and then the other, to reveal any deeply placed branches or tributaries (Fig. 5.17).
5. Pass around the vessel proximal and distal tapes, untied ligatures or Silastic tubing (Fig. 5.18). They may, depending on the size of the vessel, be merely drawn upon to angle and occlude the vessel, or made to encircle it so that it can be constricted.

Alternatively, control the vessel by applying non-damaging clamps or, for very small vessels, 'bulldog' clips (Fig. 5.19). In this way you can occlude and isolate a segment.

Fig. 5.17 Gently open round-nosed forceps at right angles to the artery to displace it and ensure that there is no deep branch at risk of damage.

Fig. 5.18 A Encircle the vessel proximal and distal to the site of the procedure so that you can exert traction to tighten the tubing and occlude the lumen. **B** A tape encircles the vessel. The ends are passed through rubber tubing. If the tape ends are pulled tighter and forceps clamped across the tube, the vessel is occluded.

Fig. 5.19 Control of blood vessels. The larger vessel is controlled by an arterial clamp, the smaller by a spring 'bulldog' clip.

Fig. 5.21 Any clot forming on the longitudinal suture line in **A** is unlikely to cause serious obstruction but clot forming on the circumferential suture line in **B** causes marked narrowing.

The lumen is less impinged upon by a longitudinal suture line than it is by a circumferential suture line at one point (Fig. 5.21).

INCISION

1. Avoid damaging the intima when incising veins and arteries. This may occur if you make a rough incision that penetrates to or through the back wall.
2. Diseased arteries may have loose plaques which can be dislodged; as far as possible ensure that you make the incision in a healthy segment. The scalpel blade may also dislodge the intimal coat, separating it from the media, potentially starting a dissection.
3. Having entered the vessel, enlarge the incision using Potts scissors, ensuring the deep blade does not damage the posterior wall (Fig. 5.20). Cut cleanly without removing and reintroducing the internal scissors blade, to avoid producing a ragged incision.
4. Because veins are thin-walled they usually accommodate to longitudinal or transverse incision. Large and medium-sized arteries may be opened transversely or longitudinally but smaller arteries are usually best opened longitudinally. When the vessels are closed, clot usually forms along the suture line.

VEINS – DIRECT PROCEDURES

1. Access to veins is a valuable means of obtaining venous blood for diagnostic purposes. They make valuable substitutes for arteries that are stenosed or blocked. The most common venous disease you will encounter is varicose veins, which are lengthened, dilated and with incompetent valves.
2. Before inserting a catheter that will fill the lumen and remain, place and ligate a distal ligature and leave the long thread by which to steady and manoeuvre it. Place an untied ligature proximally. You may occlude the intervening segment by gently lifting, distracting and angulating the threads. Make a longitudinal or transverse incision in a large vein. Insert the tip of the catheter (Fig. 5.22) and relax the proximal ligature to allow the catheter to pass through. Tie the second ligature around the vein and catheter to retain it.

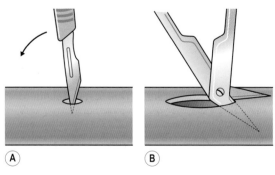

Fig. 5.20 **A** Start the incision with a pointed scalpel. **B** Extend the incision with Potts scissors.

Fig. 5.22 The vein has been tied off behind the catheter. Apply traction with the ligature thread. The other ligature is left untied until you have introduced the catheter beyond it. Then tie the ligature around the vein and contained catheter to retain it.

3. To introduce a small catheter into a large vein without occluding the lumen, first insert a small purse-string suture, with a formed but not tightened half-hitch, around the site of insertion. Control the vein using proximal and distal tapes, loops or non-damaging clamps. Carefully make a small stab into the vein and insert the catheter (Fig. 5.23). Fully advance it by partially releasing the appropriate occlusion device. Tighten and tie the purse-string and cautiously relax the occlusion, ensuring that there is no leakage.

4. Incise small veins by lifting a small portion of the wall and cutting obliquely with scissors to raise a 'V' flap. Hold this up while slipping the fine catheter underneath it and into the lumen (Fig. 5.24).

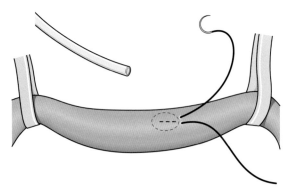

Fig. 5.23 A purse-string suture has been inserted into the vein and the straight dotted line within this indicates the site of a stab incision to accept the catheter.

Fig. 5.24 A The vein is opened obliquely to produce a 'V' flap. **B** The flap is raised so that the catheter can be inserted under it.

5. To insert a needle into an exposed very fine vein, utilize the ligatures on each side of the point of insertion to hold the vessel steady. It is sometimes an advantage to hold the needle in a gently closed needle-holder or haemostatic forceps for better control (Fig. 5.25).

Key points

- Do not allow air to enter large central veins for fear of causing air embolus to the heart and circulatory arrest.
- When tying off tributaries of main veins take great care not to narrow the main vein by applying the ligature too closely. Conversely, do not leave a cul de sac, which encourages turbulence, stagnation and consequent thrombosis (Fig. 5.26).

Varicose veins

These can be treated in a number of ways:

Intravascular sclerosants can be injected into minor veins after marking them. Approximately 1–2 mL sodium tetradecyl sulphate 1% (range 0.5–2.0%) can be injected, preferably while the leg is elevated, then bandaged. Foamed sclerosant injected under ultrasound control is claimed to be more effective. Avoid injecting near the saphenofemoral or saphenopopliteal junctions because of the risk of embolization.

Local ties are suitable for small, cosmetically important varicosities as an alternative to injection therapy. It can be performed at the time of vein stripping.

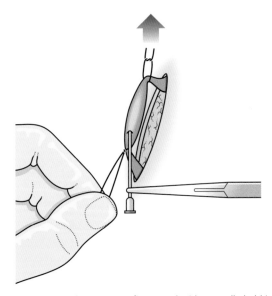

Fig. 5.25 Cannulating a very fine vessel with a needle held in a needle-holder or a haemostatic forceps.

Fig. 5.26 Tying off side branches of a large vein that will remain as a conduit or be transferred to replace or bypass an arterial block. On the left the ligature is tied too close to the main channel, constricting it. In the middle the side branch is tied off too distally, leaving a cul de sac. On the right the main channel lumen remains constant.

1. If few ties are required you may use local anaesthesia. Raise a small bleb using a fine needle. Allow sufficient time for it to act, then inject more, insinuating the needle between the vein and the overlying skin to aid the separation.
2. Make a small incision over the vein, parallel to the skin tension lines. Gently open the incision taking care not to tear the vein, then separate it from the tissues until you have encircled it. Pass a fine absorbable ligature round it, using a curved haemostat or aneurysm needle and tie it off.
3. As an alternative to ligature, you may avulse the vein after freeing it. Clamp a haemostat across it, and then rotate it on its long axis so that the vein is dragged into the wound and wrapped round the forceps, tearing the vein while maintaining pressure at the break point to prevent bleeding. Close the skin with fine absorbable stitches or adherent strips.

> **Key point**
>
> - Before operating on varicose veins ensure that you have performed the appropriate tests, that you are thoroughly familiar with the anatomy, and that the veins are carefully marked.

Saphenofemoral ligation described in 1890 by the great German surgeon from Leipzig, Friedrich Trendelenburg (1844–1924), disconnects the long saphenous system from the common femoral vein. To facilitate the procedure by emptying the leg veins he placed the patient head down, feet up – now called the 'Trendelenburg position'.

1. Through an incision placed just below the groin crease, isolate, doubly ligate and divide the tributaries entering the proximal long saphenous vein.
2. Now identify and clear the saphenofemoral junction. Doubly ligate the saphenous vein flush with the femoral vein; for extra safety use a suture ligature. Make sure that there is no constriction of the femoral vein (Fig. 5.26). Apply a ligature 1 cm distally. Divide the saphenous vein between the proximal double ligature and the single distal ligature.

Greater saphenous vein stripping may be carried out after completing the saphenofemoral ligation.

1. Make a small incision in the ligated lower cut end of the proximal saphenous vein through which to pass down the end of the stripper wire or plastic leader. Apply a loose ligature to control bleeding.
2. Advance the leader until you can feel it through the skin below and medial to the knee.
3. Make a small incision 6–8 cm below the knee joint, over the vein. Apply two untied ligatures.
4. Withdraw the end of the stripper above the lower ligature, which can then be tied. Loosely tie the upper ligature around the guidewire above the tip. Now transect the vein above the first ligature, leaving the end of the guidewire projecting from the upper cut end. Gently draw on the guidewire until the stripper head is close against the upper free end of the vein.
5. Elevate the limb, and if possible, apply compression bandages. In a controlled fashion, draw the guidewire down to strip out and concertina the vein until it emerges at the below knee incision (Fig. 5.27). This is inversion stripping of the vein.
6. Squeeze out the blood by 'milking' it along the track of the stripped vein. Roll a sterile crepe bandage from the start point progressively towards the extraction wound.
7. Finally, close the incisions.
8. An alternative is to pass the stripper from below upwards – this obviates the possible difficulty of obstruction by the valves to the passage of the stripper.

Endovenous ablation can be performed through a catheter passed from the ankle or knee up to the saphenofemoral junction, confirmed by visible light and ultrasound imaging. Endoluminal radiofrequency, laser or high-frequency ultrasound heat and energy source is now activated as the catheter is slowly withdrawn, to coagulate the vein. Ablation can be achieved under local anaesthetic by first injecting 200 mL low-dose local anaesthetic around the vein as a heat sink.

Arterial replacement with vein

Vein is frequently used as a conduit for diseased peripheral and coronary arteries.

Fig. 5.27 Principles of vein stripping. **A** After transecting the vein on the left, pass the leader through the vein. On the right the vein has again been transected so that the leader can emerge and be brought out of the wound. **B** After ensuring that the stripper head lies safely in the subcutaneous tissues, exert traction on the leader in a controlled manner, drawing it to the right. **C** The segment of vein emerges, concertina'd on the stripper.

1. A length of vein is harvested, the tributaries are tied off, avoiding narrowing. The vein is reversed so the valves do not obstruct the flow, and it can now be used as a bypass graft.
2. It is important to handle the vein gently, avoid over-distending it and preserve the adventitia around it to minimize the likelihood of it developing spasm.[1]

Key points

- Damage caused by unrecognized overdistension is a cardinal cause of failure.
- Separation of endothelial cells exposes the subepithelium to platelet adhesion.
- It is one of the factors that make the difference between the success of one surgeon and the failure of another, even though they appear to have carried out the same manoeuvre.
- Keep it in mind when you are tempted to treat the tissues roughly.

---

3. Alternatively, in the leg a segment of saphenous vein can be used in situ after passing a special instrument (a valvulotome) to destroy the valves and united to the artery above and below the occlusion to bypass it.

ARTERIES – DIRECT PROCEDURES

During arterial procedures it may be necessary to inject or apply local topical heparin; in this case make up 500 mL isotonic saline containing 5000 international units (IU) to instil locally.

Incision and closure

1. First isolate the artery and obtain control using encircling tapes, untied ligatures, Silastic tubing, or placed but not tightened clamps.

2. Longitudinal incision and closure is usually suitable for medium-sized arteries but would seriously narrow smaller vessels, since eversion of the edges to obtain intimal contact increases the narrowing. Large vessels can be incised longitudinally and transversely without seriously narrowing them.

Direct catheterization

The exposed, intact artery can be cannulated or catheterized directly, either proximally or distally. First ensure that you have proximal and distal control. A wide-bore artery may be opened transversely but use a longitudinal incision for a narrow vessel. Insert the tip of the catheter and relax the controlling tape, tube or clamp while fully advancing the catheter.

Embolectomy

This is typically performed by direct insertion of a balloon catheter, invented by the American surgeon Fogarty (while he was still a medical student), to remove an embolus or clot, for example, lodged in a peripheral artery.

1. Fully heparinize the patient with systemic heparin, 70 units/kg.
2. Control the vessel proximally and distally. Pass the catheter first proximally and then distally and withdraw it after gently inflating the balloon to fill the lumen and act as an extractor. As the catheterization is extended distally, use finer catheters.
3. Inject heparin in saline into the cleared vessels, prior to suturing the arteriotomy and releasing the clamps or tapes.

Vein patch

This offers a valuable means of avoiding serious narrowing of the lumen when closing a longitudinal incision in an artery. The patch must smoothly and slightly enlarge the diameter of the vessel. If it is too small it will not have achieved its aim. If it is too big it will so enlarge the lumen as to cause turbulence and possibly result in local thrombus formation and intimal hyperplasia. If you use saphenous vein select a proximal segment which better withstands the higher arterial pressure.

1. Excise a suitable segment of peripheral vein just longer than the defect and split it longitudinally to form a flat sheet. Trim one end to form a rounded ellipse that will fit into one end of the incision. Take a double-needled suture of suitable size and insert both needles side by side through the elliptical cut end of the graft from outside into the lumen (Fig. 5.28). Bring them from inside to the outside, just beyond and on each side of one end of the incision, so that the suture is halved. When the suture is tied it initiates an everting effect.

2. Continue from here, taking one suture along the back wall, one on the front wall as continuous over-and-over sutures. Each stitch passes in through the patch, out through the arterial wall. On the back wall you may need to suture from near to far; as a beginner be willing to change sides in order to sew from far to near. The flexibility of the vein patch makes it relatively easy to ensure that there is sufficient eversion to achieve intimal contact. As you reach the half-way point, leave the sutures on either side, while ensuring that the tension on them is not slackened, and direct your attention to the open end.

3. Trim the end of the vein patch into a rounded ellipse to fit into the remaining defect. Carry on inserting sutures on the back wall until you have rounded the end and continue on to meet the anterior wall sutures. As the stitching is completed, both sutures emerge on the arterial surface and if adjacent sutures are tied together, they form an everting mattress suture. Do not insert sutures in such a manner that at the end you cannot be sure that the stitches have picked up the endothelium. If necessary, have the tension maintained up to a point about 1 cm before you reach the stitch from the other end. Insert the last three or four stitches slackly, under direct view. Now you can tighten them seriatim to the correct tension, and confidently tie the thread to that inserted from the other end.

4. An alternative method is to start on the anterior wall near one end, with a simple running stitch and proceed around the corner onto the back wall. Continue along the back wall, trim the patch and carry the suture around the second corner, back onto the anterior wall. Insert stitches along this wall until you reach the starting stitch and tie off.

> **Key point**
>
> - Avoid finishing and tying the sutures at the end of an ellipse.

ARTERIAL ANASTOMOSIS

End-to-end anastomosis

A circular suture line results in some narrowing. This can be overcome by cutting the ends obliquely (see Fig. 5.33). Any clot that forms on a transverse suture line impinges on the lumen through its whole circumference (Fig. 5.21).

Fig. 5.28 Inserting a vein patch. **A** Excise a segment of peripheral vein. **B** Split it longitudinally. **C** Open it out. **D** Trim one end into a rounded ellipse. **E** Insert stitches in the patch and into the end of the arterial incision. **F** Continue round, keeping ahead on the back wall. Trim the end to fit into the remaining defect. **G** Carry the back wall suture around the end and continue to join the anterior suture, and tie them off.

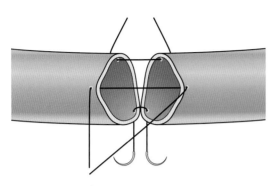

Fig. 5.29 Triangulation method of vascular anastomosis – Carrel manoeuvre.

1. When joining two arteries of equal diameter end-to-end, you can usually rotate the vessels, so enabling you to suture the circumference totally from the outside by taking one third at a time. Insert stay stitches between the two ends at one third of the circumference intervals (Fig. 5.29). This manoeuvre was devised by the French founder of vascular surgery, Alexis Carrel (1873–1944), who won the Nobel prize in 1912. By picking up two of the three sutures and slightly distracting them, the intervening edges are brought together and straightened, to facilitate stitching.
2. Begin by rotating the vessels in order to insert the first of a series of sutures, starting at the most inaccessible posterior part. Work on both sides to come round towards the anterior surface, using the traction stitches to rotate the vessels.
3. Use unlocked stitches – they form a spiral around the circumference; because the suture is smooth and unlocked, it can accommodate to arterial pulsatile distension. As the artery distends the suture tightens, reducing the tendency for leakage at the anastomosis.
4. For small vessels and in children, use interrupted stitches. In children the continuous spiral restricts arterial growth in diameter.
5. Place and tie each stitch as though you will not be able to approach it subsequently. Take care to achieve intimal contact for every stitch. Insert the stitches from outside to inside on the upstream side, from inside out on the downstream side (Fig. 5.30). If the intima is separated on the upstream side it will separate only to the anastomosis. If it is lifted on the downstream edge the dissection may spread distally.
6. The interval between stitches depends on the size of the vessels but for medium-sized arteries place them 2–3 mm apart and inserted 2–3 mm from the edges.
7. Aim to finish on the superficial face and insert the last few stitches before tying them, while ensuring that the intima is caught on each side. Only then

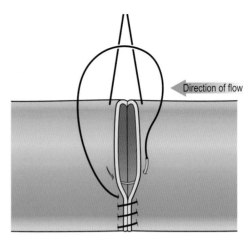

Fig. 5.30 When suturing an end-to-end anastomosis with a continuous running or interrupted stitch, insert the needle from without in on the upstream side, from within out on the downstream side.

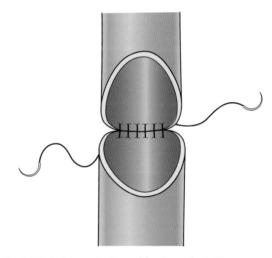

Fig. 5.31 End-to-end suture of fixed vessels starting on the back wall, identifying and picking up the full thickness including the intima in every stitch, and working towards the front.

carefully tighten them seriatim, using a nerve hook if necessary. When you are sure that every suture is perfectly placed, carefully tie them.
8. If it is not possible to mobilize and rotate the arterial ends, first insert the posterior stitches under direct vision (Fig. 5.31).
9. If necessary, leave the vessels apart, use a continuous, unlocked, double-needled suture then tighten the stitches seriatim, starting with the posterior central stitch and working outwards alternately on each side, towards the most recently inserted ones, then continue round to the front. Ensure that every one has a perfect

Fig. 5.32 Continuous suture anastomosis using the 'parachute' technique of placing the back wall sutures while the ends lie at a distance, then tightening the threads to bring the ends together.

grasp of the intima. This is the 'parachute' technique (Fig. 5.32). You can then continue on to the sides until the suture lines meet at the front.

10. In some situations it is valuable to cut each end obliquely (Fig. 5.33), carrying the suture line partially along the vessels, so that the incursion of the suture line into the lumen is less localized.

End-to-side anastomosis

When joining arteries, take care to avoid narrowing the lumen and also aim to reduce turbulence to a minimum. One method to achieve this is to make the anastomosis oblique, not at right angles, and also, to make the anastomosis about twice the length of the arterial diameter.

1. Cut a longitudinal opening in the recipient artery approximately twice the length of its diameter. Slit the end of the tributary artery to open it, and shape it to fit the opening in the main artery (Fig. 5.34).

2. Insert both needles of a double-needled suture from outside in on the tributary 'heel' to inside out on the heel of the recipient. Proceed from here on both sides towards the toe. Prefer to insert stitches on the posterior wall first so that you can view the internal suture and ensure that it picks up the intima every time, before commencing the anterior stitching. Stop when you have reached the half-way point towards the toe on the posterior and anterior walls.

3. Trim the toe of the tributary vessel to fit the remaining defect.

4. Now insert a double-needled stitch with both needles passing from outside to inside, just posterior to the end of the toe and from inside to outside in the corresponding end of the longitudinal hole in the recipient. Insert, with great care, the sutures around the extremity of the toe under vision. Suture the posterior wall up to the sutures running from the heel and tie the posterior suture, then complete the anastomosis along the front wall.

> **Key point**
>
> • The critical points are at the heel and toe.

MICROVASCULAR SURGERY

Take every opportunity to gain experience with magnification techniques. Over the years the instruments, materials and success rate for vascular surgical operations have all improved. The instruments have become more delicate, the suture materials and needles have become finer and smoother, and the techniques have been refined. As a result vascular surgeons can confidently operate on smaller and smaller vessels. The trend will undoubtedly continue.

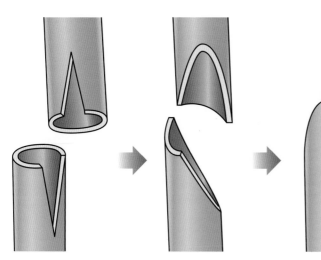

Fig. 5.33 Two small vessels are united after slitting the ends and opening them out to create a wide anastomosis.

Fig. 5.34 A small vessel has been slit before joining it into the side of another vessel. The first stitch, a double-needled thread, unites the graft to the proximal opening in the recipient vessel. Unite the graft toe to the distal end of the opening with a second double-needled thread. The back edges are first united. Stitch from each end so the back wall stitches from each end meet in the middle. Stitch the anterior wall in a similar manner.

You do not need to undertake microsurgery to benefit from acquiring the techniques. They demonstrate a level of gentle tissue handling and perfect apposition that can be transferred to the generality of surgery.

When you have the opportunity, examine a standard vascular anastomosis using magnification. What looked very neat is likely to appear coarsely fashioned.

Basic technique

1. The simplest form of magnification is a loupe (a French word with two disparate meanings – a knob, or a magnifying glass). It may be fitted to a spectacle frame (Fig. 5.35). Try the effect of performing a procedure naked eye and compare it with a similar

Fig. 5.35 A loupe fitting onto a spectacle frame provides you with magnified central vision and wide normal peripheral vision.

one carried out while wearing the loupe. You will be impressed by the greater accuracy you achieve with magnification.

2. Higher magnification is achieved using an operating microscope (Fig. 5.36). Ordinary instruments appear

Fig. 5.36 Binocular operating microscope provides shadowless illumination. Operator and assistant can view simultaneously.

Fig. 5.37 Microsurgical instruments. **A** Scissors. **B** Dissecting forceps. **C** Needle-holder. **D** Vascular clamp.

crude using this, so special instruments have been devised (Fig. 5.37).

3. Blood vessels of 1 mm diameter or less can be anastomosed with nearly 100% success. They are conveniently held in apposition using gentle microvascular clamps (Fig. 5.38). Dissect off a cuff of adventitia since any tags falling into the lumen attract platelets and provoke thrombosis (Fig. 5.39).

Fig. 5.39 Trim back the adventitia.

Fig. 5.38 Bring the vessel ends together, held by the double clamp.

Intimal damage inevitably generates clotting. Never grasp it with forceps; instead manipulate the vessels by grasping the media. You cannot produce eversion, so join the vessels end-to-end. Insert a suture through the anterior wall, ensuring that it does not pick up the posterior wall. Pick up the other anterior wall and tie the suture just to appose but not constrict or distort the continuity (Fig. 5.40). Use interrupted sutures. Space stitches every 0.3 mm in arteries, 0.6 mm in veins, with three or four on each side. After completing the anterior wall, flip over the clamp to expose what had been the posterior wall and repeat the procedure. Irrigate the vessel throughout with heparin in normal saline or Ringer's solution (Sidney Ringer 1835–1910 was an English physiologist), 1000 units in 100 mL.

101

Fig. 5.40 Penetrate the vessel wall on one side from without in and on the other pass from within out, ready to tie the suture apposing the two edges.

When the anastomosis is complete you may irrigate it with 0.5% bupivacaine. Remove the distal clamp, then the proximal clamp. Gently lift the vessel, slightly obstructing it and watch for a 'flicker' as blood flows across the constriction, confirming the patency. Apply local, gentle pressure for a few minutes if there is a leak. Occasionally you will need to insert an extra stitch after reclamping the vessel and washing out any blood adhering to the edges.

4. If you wish to create an end-to-side anastomosis, excise an ellipse in the side of the recipient vessel one third wider than the end of the vessel that will enter it.

5. Nerves can be accurately united using similar microsurgical techniques; fallopian tubes and vasa deferens can be reconstructed in a similar manner.

Key point

- If there is no flow, remove a couple of stitches, carefully wash out any clot and re-suture it. If there is still no flow, carefully excise the ends and start again.

REFERENCE

1. de Souza DSR, Pinheiro BB. Advantages of harvesting the saphenous vein for coronary artery bypass surgery using the 'no touch' technique. In: Abraham D, Handler C, Dashwood M, Coghlan G, eds. *Vascular complications in human disease*. London: Springer-Verlag; 2008:150–157.

Chapter | 6 |

Handling skin

Skin is often referred to as our largest organ. It is our interface with the outer world. Among its many functions are protection from trauma and pathogens, temperature control and sensory appreciation, the sense of touch being particularly specialized on the palmar surface of the fingers. It varies in thickness in different parts.

STRUCTURE

1. The epidermis (G *epi* = upon + *dermatos* = skin), up to 1 mm thick, consists of a basal layer producing keratinocyte daughter cells which progressively lose their DNA and become keratinized (G *keratos* = horn), squamous (L *squama* = a scale). Cell life is estimated as average 27 days before the surface cells are shed; turnover is rapid, being estimated at 4 million cells per minute in some conditions such as inflammation and psoriasis. There are no blood vessels within the epidermis.

2. The dermis contains blood vessels, nerve receptors, sweat and sebaceous glands and hairs. The papillary layer lies beneath the ridged epidermal basal layer and where these are prominent, as on the finger palms, they form friction ridges corresponding to 'finger prints'. The deeper layer is reticular (L *rete* = net) formed from interlacing connective tissue.

3. In most parts of the body skin blood supply is from the underlying muscle, vessels crossing the subcutaneous fat and forming loops at the junction with the reticular dermis, supplying the capillary network. Composite blocks of tissue are supplied by the same source artery, each block being called,

Sebaceous gland
Erector pili muscle
Sweat gland

Epidermis
Thin split-skin graft
Thick split-skin graft
Lower border of dermis
Subcutaneous fat

Fig. 6.1 Structure of skin showing epidermis and dermis. Note the levels, indicated on the right, at which to cut a thin or thick split-skin graft. The arterial supply is from the deep vessels directly or through deep structures such as muscles. They form angiosomes (see text) with linking small calibre 'choke' vessels.

Fig. 6.2 Tension lines tend to run parallel to the creases seen at joints.

by analogy with dermatomes, an 'angiosome'. The angiosome arteries are linked by small calibre 'choke' arteries that can open up to equalize the skin supply (Fig. 6.1). Likewise the matching veins are unvalved, allowing blood to flow in either direction. Mobile skin is supplied by a few large arteries, tethered skin by small dense vessels. The vessels are controlled by the autonomic system and shunts may bypass the dermis, notably in the ears, nose and fingertips.

4. Skin is unforgiving if it is overstretched, crushed, deprived of blood supply, or irradiated. Elasticity gradually disappears in old age and disease. The underlying orientation of the dermal fibrous tissues produces lines of skin tension identified by the Viennese anatomist Carl Langer (1819–1987). They usually run circumferentially around joint lines (Fig. 6.2). On the face they run at right angles to subcutaneous muscles and can be identified by asking the patient to grimace. Particularly on the face try to detect the relaxed skin tension lines that follow the furrows of the relaxed skin, detected by pinching a fold; they often follow the line between prominent underlying bones. Incisions made and closed along these lines heal with less distortion and scarring than those made across the lines of tension.

5. Skin vitality is often difficult to judge by inspection. Viability in skin flaps can be assessed by administering sodium fluorescein intravenously and the perfusion rate measured with a surface fluorometer. Until we know all the factors involved, and how they interact, it is not always possible to predict the outcome following an injury, operation or disease process. Plastic surgeons have accumulated a great deal of practical experience of value to the generality of surgeons who need to cross the skin barrier to deal with their own special system of expertise. Take every opportunity to watch and learn from them.

HEALING

Open wounds

1. Healing is achieved through a complex serious of overlapping developments.
2. Initially, haemostasis is achieved by platelet adherence to the exposed vascular subepithelium, plugging it, followed by the sequence of conversion of fibrinogen to fibrin resulting in thrombosis. Inflammation is generated by many factors including bradykinin (G *bradus* = slow + *kinin* = to move), creating vasodilatation and loss of endothelial cell contact, with increasing permeability of vessels. Inflammatory cells are attracted to the area, where neutrophils remove debris, as do monocytes, some of which convert to macrophages. These also secrete growth factors attracting endothelial cells, fibroblasts and epithelial keratinocytes. Cellular proliferation starts with the laying down of a provisional extracellular matrix (G *mater* = mother; womb, ground-mass or skeleton in or on which anything is developed). The complex matrix is composed of numerous molecules including fibronectin (L *nectere* = to bind) and hyaluronidase. This complex extracellular membrane is not a mere inert skeleton but involves integrins – adhesion molecules controlling attachment of cells to it and to each other, and ligands which bind to receptors and alter function. The provisional extracellular membrane facilitates cell migration and is gradually replaced with collagen.
3. A number of influences, including vascular endothelial growth factor, stimulate endothelial cells to migrate and form capillary blood vessel loops, resulting in

granulation tissue. Healthy granulation tissue forms a good base on which keratinocytes can migrate and on which skin grafts can be placed. Among the fibroblasts which accompany the new capillaries so formed are myofibroblasts containing smooth muscle actin and cytoplasmic microtubules which draw the wound edges centripetally. This is wound contraction. It can be prevented by applying a skin graft.

> **Key points**
>
> - Wound contraction provides a natural method of closing wounds.
> - Wound contracture, from the maturing and shortening of collagen formed as a scar, often results in loss of function.

4. Epithelialization results as the daughter cells of basal cells flatten and migrate across the granulation tissue, guided by cell adhesion glycoproteins and with fibroblasts laying down a basement membrane.
5. Remodelling occurs over a prolonged period after wound healing.
6. Intensive investigation is underway of fetal wound healing in which regeneration of epidermis and dermis occurs without scarring. Many differences from adult healing have been identified including the influence of many cytokines (G *kytos* = vessel, cell + *kinein* = to move), small protein molecules acting as intercellular mediators. An important one is transforming growth factor-β released by platelets, which promotes the laying down of an extracellular matrix and influences fibroblast proliferation.
7. The influence of extracellular matrix is being extensively studied. Preparations as sheets and powder applied to wounds are claimed to influence the regeneration and reconstruction of tissues instead of scar repair.

WOUND MANAGEMENT

1. A wound (Ger *Wunde*) is an open injury. From the history of the injury, sedulous clinical examination, and if necessary from appropriate imaging, assess the damage before starting the repair. Determine whether there is coincident damage to nerves, vessels, bones, tendons and soft tissues; in penetrating injuries, look for exit wounds. Do not, though, blindly explore the wound if you intend to open it up at operation, for fear of causing further injury.
2. Remember that many injuries have legal, compensation and insurance implications, so immediately make careful notes, drawings and photographs if possible.

3. Under sterile conditions carefully, and if necessary, widely, clean and prepare the area.
4. Explore the wound with fingers and probes, extending it when appropriate.
5. Completely stop bleeding.
6. Assiduously clean the wound. Irrigate it with plenty of sterile saline. In the presence of contamination, use only mild, aqueous-based antiseptics; strong ones damage the tissues. Take time to remove all the dead and foreign material. If you leave ingrained dirt, healing is severely prejudiced.
7. Search for and remove all foreign material and dead tissue. Do not leave dead muscle; recognize it as being soggy and homogenized, it does not bleed when cut and does not contract when gently pinched with forceps or electrically stimulated.
8. Search for and identify deeper damage to vessels, nerves, bones and joints. Do not hesitate to enlarge the incision in these circumstances. If you do need to extend the wound in a cosmetically important area, consider following the tension lines. Carry out appropriate repair of deep tissues before deciding whether or not to close the skin.
9. Finally recheck haemostasis, repeat the irrigation of the tissues and once more check for foreign material and dead or ischaemic tissue.
10. Do not close the wound if swelling has produced tension. You may be able to reduce swelling within a limb by first elevating it for 24 hours.
11. Unless the wound is clean, tidy, looks healthy and has recently been acquired, do not close it. Leave it open and determine to carry out delayed primary closure when it appears healthy. It is difficult to assess tissue perfusion and viability by appearance; the oxygen tension beneath a closed wound falls rapidly but is at atmospheric levels if the wound is left open.[1] If there is skin loss, loosely maintain the tissues in their correct position and defer attempts at reconstruction. If you are experienced you may cover a clean wound with a split-skin graft (see later).
12. If it is safe to close the wound but it is irregular and sited in a cosmetically important place such as the face, take the greatest care to align the skin correctly to avoid producing a distorted scar.

> **Key points**
>
> - Do not attempt immediate primary closure of doubtful wounds.
> - In the presence of delayed presentation, trauma, contamination, foreign material or ischaemia and tissue loss, be prepared to monitor the wound for 24–48 hours to allow you to exclude infection or impending necrosis, allow oedema to settle, then carry out delayed primary closure.
> - Do not attempt to close the wound under tension.

Wound closure

1. The aim of closure is to appose the tissues in layers without tension or compression. The progressively complex steps of reconstruction are:
   a. primary closure – suture
   b. secondary closure/delayed primary closure (secondary intention)
   c. local flap
   d. distant flap
   e. free flap.
2. Provided you cause minimal trauma, and achieve perfect haemostasis, the risks of haematoma, inflammation and infection are reduced.
3. The result is rapid linking across the wound by fibroblasts and rapid healing with minimal scarring.
4. Secondary closure is spontaneous skin closure by a combination of wound contraction and re-epithelialization. In the case of extensive skin loss, scar tissue is laid down and contracts as it matures, drawing in skin from the area, often resulting in loss of function. Continuous remodelling takes place while a defect exists and also after healing has occurred.
5. Closure with a graft or flap is sometimes referred to as tertiary closure.
6. The healing of some wounds is claimed to be helped by vacuum-assisted closure. The wound is filled with a foam substance. A drainage tube is inserted into, or laid on, the foam and the part is then covered with impermeable film. Suction is applied at around 125 mmHg between dressing changes (see Ch. 11). The wide variety of acute, traumatic, chronic, diabetic, ischaemic and infective wounds makes it difficult to assess the benefits.

ANALGESIA

(G *an* = not + *algein* = to feel pain.)

1. If local anaesthesia is unlikely to suffice on its own, consider, as an alternative to general anaesthesia, giving premedication with systemic analgesics – but this is appropriate only if you have full facilities for resuscitation and postoperative recovery.
2. Always have adrenaline (epinephrine) 1:1000 and hydrocortisone 100 mg available in case the patient develops an allergic or other reaction.
3. Lidocaine (lignocaine) and prilocaine in a concentration of 4% is effective when applied topically on mucous membranes but is ineffective on the skin. However, consider applying it topically into open wounds or serous cavities, joint spaces and fracture sites. Lidocaine 25 mg and prilocaine 25 mg in 1 g of cream (EMLA®) applied 1.5–3 g/cm² for a minimum of 2 hours under an occlusive dressing is usually effective in producing skin analgesia.

4. Local infiltration anaesthesia is a simple and safe method of producing a limited area of analgesia. Lidocaine 0.5–2.0% can be injected up to a maximum of 3 mg/kg body weight and its effect lasts up to 90 minutes. A maximum of 7 mg/kg can be injected with 1:200 000 adrenaline to cause vasoconstriction, reducing bleeding and slowing absorption. Bupivacaine injected in concentrations of up to 0.5% with a maximum dose of 2 mg/kg body weight produces up to 12 hours of analgesia. It takes several minutes to take effect; lidocaine 1% and bupivacaine 0.5% may be mixed in equal volumes to overcome this. Ropivacaine 0.75% may be safer than bupivacaine.
5. First raise an intracutaneous bleb, using a fine needle, away from a sensitive or inflamed area. Mark or note the place because the bleb will be absorbed and disappear. Wait for it to take effect, then inject through the anaesthetized spot, along the line of the proposed incision. You may produce a raised ridge resembling orange peel. Now infiltrate deeper, using a longer and larger needle, keeping the point moving as you inject, to minimize the danger of injecting into a vein.
6. Do not inject under high pressure, especially in the presence of inflammation. It is painful and the pressure of fluid will restrict the blood supply, as will the addition of adrenaline. A notorious risk when infiltrating a ring of local anaesthetic around the base of a finger is to raise the circumferential pressure and may result in finger necrosis. Always inject proximally at the level of the interphalangeal web. The risk can be further reduced by adding 1500 units of hyaluronidase, which aids the rapid spread of the anaesthetic within the tissues.

Key points

- Do not begin the procedure until the anaesthetic has had time to act. Wait a minimum of 4–5 minutes.
- You undermine the confidence and trust of the patient if your initial act causes pain.

INCISION

1. Decide the line and depth of the incision, taking into account the primary purpose of the procedure but secondarily considering the cosmetic effects, including the direction of the tension lines. If the incision will be complicated, first mark matching points with skin ink or 'Bonney's blue' dye (Victor Bonney, London gynaecologist 1872–1953) so that you can accurately appose them during closure.

Fig. 6.3 Steady the skin using the fingers and thumb of your non-dominant hand.

2. Stretch and fix the skin at the starting point using your non-dominant hand (Fig. 6.3).
3. Except when creating a short stab wound, use the belly of the knife and draw it along the line of the incision, rather than pressing it in statically. Cut to an even depth throughout so that you can use the whole length of the wound. Do not leave half incised ends that add to the length of the scar and add nothing to the access.
4. When possible cut boldly with a single sweep of the knife. Tentative scratches detach pieces that will undergo necrosis and delay healing (Fig. 6.4). Occasionally scissors are preferable to a scalpel for cutting loose flaps provided the blades are rigid and remain in contact; if they separate, the skin will be crushed and 'chewed'. Cut perpendicular to the surface to avoid slicing it.
5. Control initial oozing from the cut edges by pressing with your fingertips along one edge while your assistant presses on the opposite side (Fig. 6.5). Use folded gauze swabs if necessary. Diminish severe oozing by applying haemostatic forceps at intervals of about 1 cm, to the dermal edges – not the epidermis – and lay the forceps handles onto the intact surface to evert the edges (Fig. 6.6). Never place haemostatic forceps on the epidermis. This crushes the skin and produces ugly scarring. The least damaging method is to retract the edges using fine skin hooks. You may identify and pick up individual vessels with fine artery forceps, twist them and release them. Avoid

Fig. 6.4 Make smooth incisions, as illustrated in **A**. Multiple cuts produce ragged incisions (**B**) with tags that will die and delay healing.

Fig. 6.5 Reduce oozing by compressing one edge with your non-dominant fingers while your assistant compresses the other side. You may spread the pressure with a flattened swab.

Fig. 6.6 Control bleeding from the wound edge, especially on the scalp, by attaching haemostatic forceps to the dermis and using them to evert the skin. However, hand-held skin hooks are less damaging.

ligatures close to the skin surface. Use diathermy current sparingly since skin burns heal slowly; pick up the vessel with fine forceps, apply 'cutting' current at the lowest intensity for the minimal time. Bipolar diathermy is safer than monopolar diathermy, since the current passes only between the two forceps tips and does not heat surrounding tissues.

EXCISION

Skin lesions

1. Many lesions are amenable to excision under local anaesthesia. In the absence of infection, tend to use a dilute solution, with added adrenaline, that can be infiltrated widely over the extent of the lesion, to reduce oozing.

2. When excising skin that is diseased, scarred, traumatized, ischaemic or adherent to a lesion that must be completely excised, plan it carefully, if necessary marking the incision with skin ink or Bonney's blue dye. Take into account the site – facial skin has an excellent blood supply and heals well, palmar skin of the hands and plantar skin of the feet is specialized and cannot be replaced with skin of equal quality and nerve supply. Elderly patients often have mobile spare skin.

3. When excising circular lesions plan an elliptical incision, aligned with the tension lines, with pointed ends (Fig. 6.7). The wider the ellipse, the longer it should be, otherwise the resulting scar will be ugly.

4. Excise benign lesions within the skin allowing minimal margins. There is no need to remove deep tissue.

5. Subcutaneous benign lesions attached to the skin may need to be excised with an ellipse of the involved skin. The specimen resembles a boat.

6. A malignant lesion should be totally excised with a margin of normal skin. In particular, *malignant melanoma* must be treated expertly. Its local invasiveness is measured by the Clark's level – the depth of infiltration. The most reliable prognostic measurement is the Breslow thickness from the granular layer of skin to the deepest growth. If the depth is less than 2 mm, a margin of normal skin of 1 cm appears to be safe but if it is greater than 2 mm a wider margin appears to be necessary. The incision should be carried vertically down to the deep fascia. The prognostic benefit of sentinel node biopsy (see Ch. 7) in malignant melanoma is not yet defined but as results are collected it is likely that the indications for, and impact on further management, will be clarified.[2]

7. Make the incision while keeping the scalpel blade perpendicular to the skin surface to avoid slicing it. In some areas, such as the skin near the eyelids of young people, this may cause distortion and a local flap may provide a better cosmetic result.

Intradermal or subcutaneous cyst

1. This can be excised under local anaesthesia. You rarely need to shave the hair.

2. Carefully raise an intracutaneous bleb at the edge of the swelling. Through this inject dilute (0.5%) lidocaine intracutaneously over the top and around

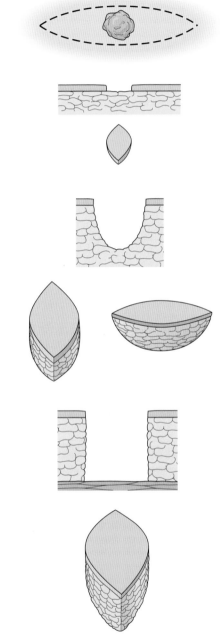

Fig. 6.7 Elliptical excision of lesions of the skin or attached to the skin. Above is shown the elliptical shape enclosing the lesion. It is preferably parallel to the skin tension lines. Below this is shown the horizontal defect resulting after removing a superficial skin lesion, with the specimen below it. Below this is shown the defect resulting from the excision of a lesion extending into the subcutaneous tissues, with below it, the boat-shaped specimen. At the bottom is shown the defect following the excision of a possible or likely malignant melanoma, and the specimen with vertical walls extending down to the deep fascia.

but not into the cyst. The volume of anaesthetic separates the cyst from the surrounding tissues.

3. Do not rush to make the incision. Allow about 5 minutes for the local anaesthetic to take effect.

4. Place the incision just off centre of the punctum or summit of the swelling, otherwise you risk entering the cyst.

5. Achieve haemostasis by identifying the small intradermal vessels and catching them with fine haemostats. The vessels lie in the subcuticular layer, not in the epithelium, so avoid catching this. As a rule, it is sufficient to leave on the haemostats until you are ready to close, but one or two vessels may need to be ligated with the finest absorbable material. If you intend to use diathermy coagulation, set it at the lowest effective setting and use it for the minimum time. If you burn the epithelium it will produce a visible scar. Prefer bipolar current diathermy.

6. Identify the cyst wall, work around it and gradually free it without rupturing it. Avoid grasping it with forceps. The last portion to free should be the punctum, attached to the skin surface; if necessary excise a small ellipse with it, to avoid puncturing it.

7. If you rupture the cyst, carefully identify all the lining and excise it to prevent a recurrence.

8. After securing haemostasis, suture the skin.

9. As an alternative to a dressing, apply a varnish skin spray.

CLOSURE

Simple linear

1. Close a simple incision by accurately re-apposing the living skin edges. To avoid any displacement of the edges of a straight incision, insert skin hooks at each end and have them gently distracted by an assistant while you insert the stitches.

2. Healing cannot take place if the dead, keratinized surface cells are apposed by inverting the edges. It is preferable to err on the side of slight eversion (Fig. 6.8).

3. For many closures, insert stitches 2–3 mm from the edges, 2–3 mm deep, 2–3 mm apart. You may need to take larger or smaller bites depending on the site, and the size of the wound closure.

4. Insert stitches on curved needles held in needle-holders. Use cutting needles mounted with fine thread. Silk has for many years been the standard material but in recent years fine monofilament polyamide and polypropylene have become popular and are claimed to cause minimal tissue reaction, especially for closing wounds on the face.

5. Grip the needle in the needle-holder on the swaged side of the middle. Fully pronate your hand so that

Fig. 6.8 **A** The skin edges are inverted, achieving contact only between the dead keratinized surfaces. **B** The edges are slightly everted; the living edges are in contact and can unite.

the needle point enters perpendicular to the skin surface from the dominant side to emerge on the non-dominant side, or from the far side to near. As you progressively supinate your hand to drive the needle along the path of its curve, it emerges in the wound. Capture it and reinsert it into the other side exactly opposite. Progressively supinate your hand to drive the needle in a curved path through the tissues.

6. If the wound is in the sagittal plane in relation to you, insert the needle from your dominant to non-dominant side. Start from far away and work towards you. If the wound lies transversely, insert the suture from far to near, placing the first stitches on your non-dominant side, working towards your dominant side. This is not a firm rule. What is important is for you to feel comfortable and in control.

7. In some cases you may pass the needle across the gap, to emerge on the opposite side. In other circumstances you may need to pass through the needle on one side, capture it in the gap and reinsert it on the opposite side at a point in the same line. As the point emerges at the skin level, once more capture it, further supinating your hand to draw it through (Fig. 6.9). To aid the passage of the needle, gently apply counter pressure with closed dissecting forceps or use skin hooks to evert the skin edges.

8. If the skin has a tendency to invert, use an everting mattress stitch (Fig. 6.10).

9. As important as the insertion of the suture is the tying and placing of the knot. Tie the knot just tightly enough to appose the edges. The skin will swell slightly and if you tie it too tightly you will produce a ladder scar. Site the knot to one side of the closure.

10. Remove sutures on the face after 3–4 days, and after 7–10 days in abdominal and similar wound closures.

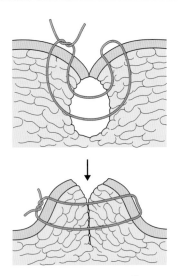

Fig. 6.10 An everting mattress suture will correct the tendency for the skin to invert.

Subcuticular stitch

1. An excellent alternative to conventional stitching is the subcuticular stitch, avoiding stitch marks on the skin. It is more difficult to ensure perfect apposition than when inserting conventional sutures. Use it only if there is no tension, or if you have overcome the tension by first inserting deeper stitches. Suitable smooth, non-absorbable material is monofilament polyamide, polypropylene or polyethylene.
2. Introduce the suture in the line of the wound about 1 cm from one end, into the extreme end of the wound. Insert stitches on alternate sides into the intradermal layer all at the same depth, each one crossing the gap at right angles to avoid distorting the skin (Fig. 6.11).

Fig. 6.9 Use a skin hook (**A**) or closed dissecting forceps (**B**) to evert the skin edges. Press closed forceps a short distance from the edge, or use them to push back the edge to produce eversion. **C** Make sure that the needle crosses between the edges at exactly the same depth. **D** If you grab the skin with forceps you will crush it and cause scarring, so either grip the dermis with dissecting forceps or used closed forceps to deform it.

Fig. 6.11 Skin closure. **A** Subcuticular stitch: when the stitch ends are distracted, the edges are drawn together. The stitch may be absorbable and can be left, or non-absorbable and can be withdrawn. **B** Provided the wound is absolutely dry you may appose the edges using adherent strips of tape.

3. At the far end, drive the stitch to emerge on the skin about 1 cm beyond the end in the line of the incision.

4. The intradermal stitches lie parallel to the skin surfaces. It is necessary to have the needle-holder exactly perpendicular to the undisturbed skin surface, in order to drive the curved needle in its jaws along a path parallel to the skin surface. Moreover, since you stitch alternately to one side, then the other, you need to change the needle to point towards and away from you with each stitch. However, if you evert the skin using a skin hook or apply pressure with closed dissecting forceps, you can distort the skin edges, allowing you to insert the needle with ease (Fig. 6.12). Do not use your fingers for fear of sustaining a needle prick.

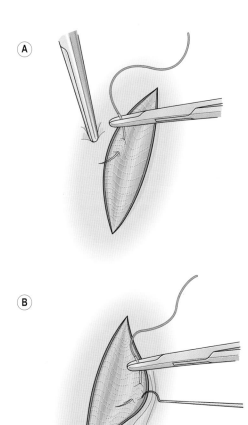

Fig. 6.12 Subcuticular stitch. By everting the skin edges you can insert stitches that will be parallel to the skin surface when the eversion is relaxed. Produce eversion either by pressing with the closed tips of dissecting forceps as shown in **A**, or traction from a skin hook as shown in **B**.

5. Having inserted all the stitches, now distract the suture ends to straighten it, thus drawing the skin edges together. Tape the ends of sutures down to the skin. When the wound is healed, release the tethering, pull each end in turn to free the thread, then cut one end flush with the skin to avoid dragging it through the wound, and pull the remainder of the intact thread out from the other end. If the wound is long there is a danger that the incision will break when you try to pull it through in one piece; to avoid this break it up into lengths of about 5–6 cm by bringing it to the surface and knotting it (Fig. 6.13).

6. Modern synthetic absorbable sutures can be inserted and do not need to be removed. Insert a subcuticular stitch at one end of the incision, picking up both sides, and tie it. Proceed from here along the wound, inserting subcuticular stitches on alternate sides until you reach the far end. You may now tie a knot after taking a stitch through both sides. This may be difficult to do. Alternatively, bring out the needle about 1 cm from the end of the wound to one side, return the needle back through the same hole to emerge within the wound. Reinsert it into the wound to emerge about 1 cm from the end on the other side and back again. Finally bring it to the surface and cut it off flush with the skin (Fig. 6.13). This offers sufficient fixation.

7. Adhesive strips also offer an alternative to conventional stitches to appose skin edges (Fig. 6.11).

Fig. 6.13 Two tips when inserting subcuticular stitches. **A** When inserting a long non-absorbable stitch, H. S. Tantawy of Cairo suggests coming to the surface every 5–6 cm, tying a slip knot, reinserting the needle into the same hole and tightening the knot down to the skin. A similar technique suffices to fix the ends. Withdraw the stitch in segments between the slip knots. **B** There are several choices for securing the ends of an absorbable subcuticular stitch. At the right end, an encircling subcuticular stitch has been inserted and tied within the wound. On the left, the needle has been brought out to the surface at an angle, and returned through the same hole; repeat this at another angle and finally bring it out and cut it flush.

Unless they adhere right up to the skin edges they have an inverting effect, so ensure there is no oozing, that the skin is completely dry. If possible, first apply an adhesive such as a plastic spray or tincture of benzoin and allow it to dry.

8. Skin staples are sometimes used as an alternative to stitches (see Ch. 2). As a trainee take every opportunity to practise stitching. It is the most versatile method of joining soft tissues. Reserve staples for exceptional circumstances when these will be of benefit to the patient.

Closing defects

1. Do not pull together skin edges under tension and expect them to heal.
2. In some cases the skin edges fail to come together, not because there is a skin deficiency but because of deficiency of the attached deep layers. You may transfer tension from the skin to the deeper layers by drawing them together first and then closing the skin without tension.
3. Close an elliptical incision (Fig. 6.14), if necessary after undermining the skin on either side. In order to appose the edges accurately it may be convenient to start in the middle, working outwards. This tends to reveal the raised 'dog ears' that may mar the appearance of the scar. Mark out the base of the dog ears and excise them so that you achieve a straight, flat scar.
4. Undercutting the skin is of value only if it is the deep attachments that prevent the edges from being drawn together (Fig. 6.15). If the skin is already tight do not expect to succeed – the freed skin edges may merely retract further. Relatively avascular skin must retain its blood supply, so include the subdermal plexus within the subcutaneous fat. Evert the skin first with dissecting forceps or a skin hook, and later with the fingers (Fig. 6.16).
5. When the lengths of the edges of a defect are incongruous, insert guide stitches that will later be removed. Place the first of these into the middle of each of the edges, and place others halving the intervening space (Fig. 6.17), and so on. Now insert the definitive stitches and then remove the guide stitches. In this way you can spread the difference in length of the edges evenly.
6. If it is important to close a defect to provide skin cover, for example over a bony fracture, it may be necessary to create a relaxing incision over a parallel area with a good blood supply in the base, so that the adjacent skin can be slid across to close the defect (Fig. 6.18). Occasionally the defect you create to close the original one needs to be closed with a skin graft.

Fig. 6.14 A A circular lesion will be excised using an elliptical incision with pointed ends as in Fig. 6.7. **B** The resulting defect. The shading indicates possible undermining of the skin edges if this will facilitate closure. **C** Close the central part first. **D** This often produces raised 'dog ears' at each end. **E** Carefully outline the bases of the dog ears and excise them as in **F**. **G** Finally close the slightly longer but flat wound.

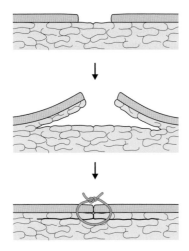

Fig. 6.15 If the skin is tethered but elastic, free it so that the edges can be apposed.

Fig. 6.16 While undercutting the skin, evert it so you keep in the right plane.

Do not embark on such a procedure unless you have special training. Inexpert management will prejudice survival of the skin cover.

7. The most generally effective temporary measure is to apply a split-skin graft.

GRAFTS

1. The name is said to arise from the fact that shoots cut for grafting trees resembled a stylus or pen with which to write (= G *graphein*). Its surgical use implies tissue that is totally freed and placed elsewhere, deriving its nourishment from the tissue bed in which it is placed.

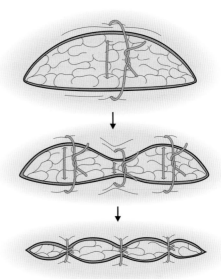

Fig. 6.17 If the length of the edges of the defect are incongruous, insert a stitch that joins the middle of each edge, then halve the space on each side and so on. When you have inserted the definitive stitches, remove the guide stitches. In this way you spread the difference in length evenly.

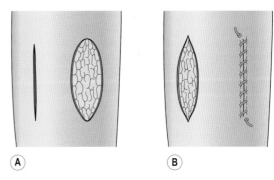

(A)　　　　　　　　　(B)

Fig. 6.18 A A defect that must be covered with good-quality skin; to the left of the defect a relaxing incision has been made. **B** The bridge of skin between the relaxing incision and the defect has been mobilized and slid across to cover the defect. The resulting gap could be closed with a split-skin graft.

2. Grafts can be cut under general or local anaesthesia. If you use local anaesthesia, consider first applying a cream containing lidocaine 25 mg and prilocaine 25 mg/g. Apply 1.5–3 g/cm² for a minimum of 2 hours beneath an occlusive dressing, over the donor area. Alternatively infiltrate the whole area with dilute (e.g. 0.25%) lidocaine with 1500 units of Hyalase.

3. Survival depends upon there being suitable conditions at the receptor site. These are:

    a. Adequate and stable contact between donor graft and recipient site. This implies that there is no separation because of graft movement, interposed necrotic or foreign material, slough, exudation, haematoma or seroma.

    b. Adequate blood supply to establish a source of nourishment. This implies no serious ischaemic or post-radiation effects at the recipient site.

    c. Absence of certain types of microorganisms, in particular β-haemolytic *Streptococcus* type A, which produces fibrinolysin, thus prejudicing adherence of the graft.

Split-skin graft

1. This general purpose graft, described by Karl Thiersch of Erlangen and Leipzig in 1874, includes some germinal layers but leaves behind the hair follicles, sebaceous glands and sweat glands, which provide fresh epithelial cells to resurface the donor area within usually 1–2 weeks.

2. Split-skin grafts may be thin, requiring minimal nourishment and therefore surviving when the blood supply is relatively poor. They are fragile and not capable of withstanding heavy wear and tear. The donor site heals rapidly, allowing the taking of further grafts – useful if extensive skin replacement is required. Thick skin grafts demand a suitable base but once established are relatively robust. The donor site heals slowly.

3. The recipient site may be fresh, as following excision of tissues including skin, or following preparation after skin loss resulting from burns, ulcers, pressure sores and other causes of skin loss.

4. Following surgical excision or traumatic skin loss, immediate skin grafting can be carried out provided the base has an adequate blood supply; fat is poorly supplied with blood vessels and makes a poor recipient base, as does bone stripped of its periosteum. Before applying a skin graft achieve absolute haemostasis, since bleeding beneath the graft prevents it from adhering to the bed and gaining nutriments.

5. Healthy granulation tissue consisting of capillary loops and fibroblasts makes a suitable recipient base. It should be pink, fairly compact and not oedematous, with minimum exudation, and no slough. Take swabs for culture. Infection with many organisms does not preclude grafting but group A β-haemolytic *Streptococcus* prevents successful graft take and it releases hyaluronic acid, which prevents graft adhesion. If slough is present, be willing to excise it surgically. Ultrasound removal of slough is sometimes recommended. If granulation tissue does not form on a raw area this suggests that a graft is unlikely to survive.

6. Cut the graft using a Watson modification of the Humby knife, which has an adjustable roller to control the thickness of the cut by adjusting the gap between the blade and the roller. As a rough guide, the no. 15 blade of a Swann-Morton disposable scalpel blade will just pass between the knife blade and the roller. A smaller instrument, the Silver knife, is valuable for cutting small grafts.

7. Grafts can be cut using powered dermatomes driven by electrical or compressed air motors. They reliably cut even grafts (Fig. 6.19). As a trainee aim to develop your skill using a hand-held knife.

8. Depending on the recipient site and the required extent of the graft, you may select the donor site. A common donor area is the upper lateral front of the thigh. You need a flat skin surface and this is created by preceding the knife blade with a lubricated flat board held in your non-dominant hand while your assistant holds a dry board, steadily applying counter pressure above the donor site to slightly stretch it and flatten it (Fig. 6.20) with one hand, while supporting the undersurface of the limb with the other hand, to create the largest and flattest area possible.

9. After adjusting the roller and lubricating the undersurface of the blade, hold the graft knife flat

Fig. 6.19 Powered dermatome.

against the skin, concentrating on smoothly drawing it back and forth in a sawing motion, as you slowly draw the board just ahead of the knife, flattening and tensing the skin so that the knife blade does not drag it back and forth without cutting it.

Key points

- Closely watch an expert cut grafts and make sure you are supervised until you become competent at this procedure.
- Do not press hard, or try to advance too quickly.
- Do not angle the knife or it will cut out.
- Try not to stop until you have completed the whole graft.

10. The graft accumulates on the knife like thin paper in folds. The donor site appears initially white, soon erupting with fine petechial haemorrhages if the graft is thin and with larger drops and more prolific bleeding following a deeper cut. Too thick a graft reveals subcutaneous fat. When you have completed the cut, raise the knife to lift the curtain-like graft and cut across with scissors.

Key points

- If you expose fat do not continue; the donor site will not heal.
- Lay the graft back on the donor site, suture it in place and move to a different site.

11. Lay a large graft on tulle gras, outer side (dull, keratinized) down, living surface (shiny, pink) uppermost. Gently open out and spread the graft using closed dissecting forceps.
12. Pick up the tulle gras with attached graft and lay it, graft side down, onto the recipient site, allowing it to overlap the edges of the defect. Make small incisions in the graft to allow for drainage.
13. A popular method of fixing the graft is to insert stitches around the periphery to fix it and use these to fix a compressing dressing over it. Insert the stitches through the graft then through the skin; if you insert it first through the skin you lift off the graft (Fig. 6.21). Leave the suture long after tying it. If you cause bleeding under the graft carefully squeeze it out and maintain compression until it stops. When the graft has been encircled with sutures place a carefully shaped cotton wool pad over the graft and tie the ends of the stitches over it to hold it in place. Plastic surgeons often use cotton wool impregnated with flavine emulsion or alternatively use shaped polyurethane sponge. Depending on the site and your

Fig. 6.20 Cutting a split-skin graft. Hold a lubricated flat board in your left hand and slowly draw it ahead of the knife held in the right hand, to flatten and stretch the skin as you cut the graft with a back and forth movement. Your assistant holds a dry, fixed board above the start of the cut to flatten, stretch and fix the skin. The assistant's other hand may lift up the soft tissues from below to expose a larger area on the upper surface.

Fig. 6.21 On the left, the needle has passed first through the skin and as it pushes up through the graft it tends to lift and displace it. On the right, the needle first passes through the graft without displacing it.

ability to attain fixation and create even compression, you may insert stitches only or compression only.
14. The donor site was formerly covered with tulle gras but alginate dressings such as Kaltostat® are more comfortable. The donor site is more painful than the recipient site.

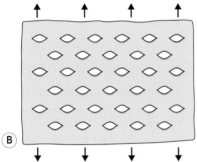

Fig. 6.22 The skin graft can be passed through a mesher which produces small cuts. You can mesh it using a scalpel. **A** Make a series of cuts in the split-skin graft. **B** The graft can be stretched to increase its area.

15. Meshed grafts have several advantages. The skin is normally fed between rollers that cut it in a pattern that allows the sheet to be extended in a net-like pattern (Fig. 6.22). If a machine is not available it is possible to create small mesh grafts using a scalpel. Meshing increases the area of the graft, valuable if there is a large defect. Its other main advantage is that any exudates, blood or pus can pass through the holes in the mesh instead of gathering under the graft and lifting it off.
16. Store any spare skin graft in the refrigerator at approximately 4°C for up to 3 weeks after being wrapped in sterile saline-moistened gauze.

Full-thickness graft

1. This was described in 1873 by John Wolfe, an Austrian ophthalmologist who settled in Glasgow. It includes all layers of the skin freed of subcutaneous tissue. Because the whole thickness of skin is used, the donor site will not heal spontaneously but may be closed after gently undermining the edges.

2. It is often used on the face because the cosmetic appearance is very good if the donor site is carefully selected for thickness and colour. Favourite donor sites for replacement facial skin include post-auricular, supraclavicular, antecubital and groin.
3. Because of its thickness the recipient site must be clean with a satisfactory vascular base and edges.
4. Make a pattern of the defect and draw it on the donor site with skin ink or Bonney's blue dye.
5. Cut the graft with perpendicular edges, avoiding slicing them. Turn the graft and carefully cut off all the fat, since this will form a partition separating the graft from the base, depriving it of nutrition.
6. Carefully sew in the graft. As it is excised it shrinks and must be slightly stretched to normal tension to fit accurately into the new site.
7. The donor site can usually be closed as a linear scar.

FLAPS

A flap, unlike a graft, retains its blood supply through a pedicle instead of picking up a fresh supply at the recipient area like a free graft.

Random pattern flaps have a haphazard blood supply. Because of this the length of the base attachment is critical in relation to the length of the flap. Many such flaps survive better if they are raised but then returned to their base for two weeks before transfer.

Axial pattern flaps were identified when it was recognized that some flaps could be much longer in relation to the base and still survive. The reason proved to be that the blood vessels remained intact entering the base of the flap. These flaps may incorporate subcutaneous fat, fascia, muscle and bone.

Free flaps are axial pattern flaps in which the supplying blood vessels are divided and are then anastomosed to vessels at another site where the graft is needed (see later).

Z-plasty

1. This overcomes the problem of linear shortening by taking advantage of the fact that skin is flexible and elastic; it may be shifted in from the side to increase the length of the contracture.
2. In Fig. 6.23 the diamond shape at the top is wider than its height. The line XY in the top diagram represents a linear contraction. Make an incision along it. At X make an incision of the same length downwards and to the right at an angle of 60°, at Y make an incision of the same length upwards and to the left at an angle of 60°.
3. Raise the flaps with tips marked A and B on to the bases marked with broken lines.

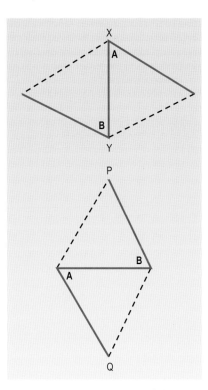

Fig. 6.23 Z-plasty. To extend the length of the line XY in the upper diagram, raise the triangular flaps marked A and B as far as the dotted lines. Transpose them and suture them in place as in the lower drawing so that the length PQ is longer than XY, at the cost of width.

4. Now transpose A anticlockwise on its base, rotate B anticlockwise on its base so that they cross as in the lower diagram. The diamond so formed is now taller than it is wide. The length PQ is greater than the height of the upper diamond, XY.
5. Increasing the angle of the side incisions increases the lengthening effect of the Z-plasty, decreasing the angle of the side incisions decreases the lengthening effect.
6. A series of Z-plasties may be used to increase the length of a long contracture by incorporating width along its whole length.

Transposition flaps

1. When skin is lost or excised it may not be possible to draw the edges together, or to do so may cause distortion. A variety of flaps may be used.
2. A simple transposition flap can be used to close a defect (Fig. 6.24). If a defect has to be closed, a suitably shaped flap can be raised and sewn in to close it.
3. Close the defect left by the flap as a linear suture line.

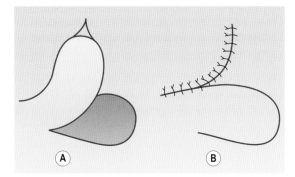

Fig. 6.24 Transposition flap. In **A** the excised area is shaded and the flap is raised. In **B** the flap has been transposed into the defect and the gap left has been closed as a linear suture line.

Myocutaneous and compound flaps

1. As understanding of the blood supply has increased, advantage has been taken especially to close skin by bringing its blood supply with it.
2. An area of skin, nourished from the underlying muscle can be moved with the body of the muscle. Many muscles, such as the latissimus dorsi, have the neurovascular bundle enter them from one end. The other end, together with an area of overlying skin can be mobilized and swung a considerable distance to fill a defect (Fig. 6.25). The latissimus dorsi flap is frequently used to restore the contour following mastectomy. An alternative is the transverse rectus

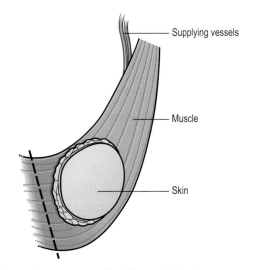

Fig. 6.25 Myocutaneous flap. The muscle has been transected along the broken line. The overlying area of skin, which derives its blood supply from the muscle, can be moved together with the muscle belly, hinging on its supplying blood vessels.

abdominis myocutaneous flap (TRAM) in which the lower rectus abdominis muscle and overlying skin are freed and swung up to the opposite breast.

3. Flaps may contain not only muscle but also fascia, cartilage and bone.

FREE TISSUE TRANSFER

Since the blood supply can be identified and preserved in an axial pattern skin flap, or to a myocutaneous flap, the vessels can be detached and the whole can be transferred elsewhere. The blood vessels are joined in to local vessels, usually two veins for each artery, employing microsurgical techniques (see Ch. 5). A popular reconstructive procedure following mastectomy is to free lower abdominal skin and fat, preserving the deep inferior epigastric perforating (DIEP) vessels and joining them to local vessels on the chest. As an alternative to the TRAM flap, this preserves the integrity of the abdominal muscles.

TISSUE EXPANSION

As an alternative to bringing in skin from elsewhere, local skin can often be obtained by expanding it. This is achieved by placing a plastic container under the fascia or muscle (Fig. 6.26). The container is connected through

Fig. 6.26 Tissue expansion. The hemispherical expander is attached to a small reservoir. The expander is inserted subfascially or submuscularly. The subcutaneously sited reservoir can be injected transcutaneously with saline to gradually distend the expander and the overlying tissues.

a connecting tube. Over a period saline can be injected into the reservoir to increase its bulk and expand the skin. When sufficient expansion has been achieved the plastic container can be removed and the spare skin is available to close a deficiency.

AESTHETIC PROCEDURES

Many procedures have been introduced to improve appearance, termed 'cosmetic' (G *kosmos* = order, *kosmein* = to adorn) or 'aesthetic' (G *aesthesthai* = feel or perceive; possessing or claiming to possess a sense of beauty).

Liposuction is the most frequently performed aesthetic procedure in the USA. A slim cannula is inserted into the subcutaneous tissue to remove excess fat. It is now usually power assisted, with infiltration of fluid such as Ringer lactate, often containing lidocaine and adrenaline. Adjunctive ultrasonic cavitation of the fat cells facilitates the removal.

Lipoplasty. Autologous fat transfer is a method of increasing contour.

Clostridium botulinum type A neurotoxin complex injections into facial muscles paralyse them, reducing wrinkles. The effect typically occurs within 3–7 days and lasts up to 4 months

Breast procedures. Following surgical operations for disease, repair and replacement may be achieved using skin grafts and flaps such as latissimus dorsi or transverse rectus abdominis myocutaneous (TRAM) (see also Ch. 7). A range of procedures are used to improve the contour. Implants are now usually of cohesive gel. Tissue expansion by, for example, a deep inferior epigastric perforating (DIEP) flap, is intended to replace or change the contour. Breast reduction may be performed to lessen the size and weight of excessively large breasts, and following a partial mastectomy for disease on one side, the other, normal breast, may be reduced to match it.

REFERENCES

1. Chang N, Goodson III WH, Gottrup F, Hunt TK. Direct measurement of wound and tissue oxygen tension in postoperative patients. *Ann Surg.* 1983;197:470–478.

2. Ariyan S. Malignant melanoma. In: Mathes SJ, ed. *Plastic surgery*. vol V. 2nd ed. Philadelphia: Elsevier; 2006:305–344.

Chapter | 7 |

Handling connective and soft tissues

Our bodies are composed of a wide variety of tissues. Some are homogeneous (G *homos* = same + *genos* = kind; made up of the same kind of cell) but most are a mixture of parenchymal cells – the soft active cells held together with connective tissue and permeated by vascular, neural and other structures. The connective tissue forms a scaffold or matrix supporting the parenchymal cells; the supportive cells are not merely passive or standardized but react with the parenchymal cells in health and disease.

Key points

- Familiarize yourself with the anatomy, structure, texture, surroundings, strength and fragility, at different ages and nutritional states, and in health and in various diseased states.
- In addition, familiarize yourself with the tissue planes between the target structure and the surrounding tissues, otherwise you risk causing inadvertent damage.

PERCUTANEOUS DIAGNOSTIC PROCEDURES

Many procedures can be carried out under local anaesthesia (see Ch. 6). The availability of ultrasound and other imaging techniques, and advanced cytological techniques enables targeted diagnostic capture of fluid, microorganisms and cells, and the introduction of, for example, radio-opaque medium, into most places within the body. Breast, thyroid and prostate glands and superficial lymph nodes, for example, are commonly investigated in this way. For deep structures, fine 'skinny' needles of 0.7 mm external and 0.5 mm internal diameter can be introduced into many organs, especially liver and lung, while respiration is temporarily suspended.

Aspiration of fluid for cytology

1. Before you insert the needle, try to confirm the exact location of the fluid by eliciting fluctuation. If not, or if the fluid lies deeply, you may use imaging methods such as ultrasound.
2. Carry out the procedure under sterile conditions. Use a needle that is long enough so you do not need to insert it to the Luer connection; otherwise, if it breaks off at the junction with the shaft, you may not be able to recapture the needle.
3. Attach a syringe and aspirate. If you obtain no fluid, try rotating the needle. Do not alter the direction of the needle except by first withdrawing it.
4. Fine-needle aspiration cytology (FNAC) can often be carried out under local anaesthetic although even this may be unnecessary. Fix the target between the fingers of one hand while holding the syringe and needle (usually a 21 gauge) in the other.
5. When the tip is correctly sited apply suction by attempting to withdraw the piston of the syringe. Move the needle in and out in jerky reciprocal movements to detach cells, which will be drawn into the needle.
6. Simultaneous fixation of a lump, control of the needle position and aspiration of a standard syringe are difficult. A number of mechanical aids are available based on the principle shown in Fig. 7.1.
7. Cell harvesting is improved if the syringe and needle are first washed out with a mixture of physiological (0.9%) saline with 1000 units of heparin. After completing the procedure, withdraw the syringe and needle and eject the contents onto several pre-labelled microscope slides and immediately apply fixative to them. Finally, draw up some fixative through the needle into the syringe from a specimen bottle and empty the syringe back into the bottle. The ejected cells will be recovered by centrifugation and stained along with those on the slides, for cytological

Fig. 7.1 The principle of fine-needle aspiration cytology. The action of a syringe holder allows the syringe and needle to be controlled with one hand while the other steadies the lump. Squeezing the handle of the syringe holder draws out the piston and exerts a suction effect through the attached needle.

examination. In some cases the cells are immediately smeared onto a slide using a cover slip, air-dried and then stained.

Needle biopsy

1. In order to confirm the histological diagnosis and grade, identify the receptor status and carry out a DNA analysis of a tumour, obtain a core of tissue. Take advice beforehand from the pathologist about how the specimen should be preserved and sent for examination.
2. If the lesion is not palpable the needle may be guided with the aid of ultrasound or radiological imaging.
3. One method is with a hollow needle such as a Trucut™ (Travenol). From the end of a sharp hollow needle protrudes the bevelled cutting end of a stylette. The proximal part of the stylette does not fill the lumen of the needle (Fig. 7.2). After infiltrating the

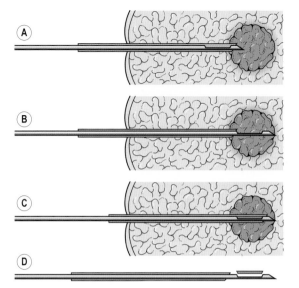

Fig. 7.2 Needle biopsy. **A** Insert the closed needle tip into the tissue that will be biopsied; **B** hold the needle still and advance the stylette into the tissue. Some of the tissue bulges against the thin shaft of the stylette; **C** hold the stylette still and advance the needle to cut off and enclose the core of tissue; **D** withdraw the needle and retrieve the core of tissue.

    skin with local anaesthetic make a small incision with a pointed scalpel, just large enough to accept the needle. Insert the closed needle through the incision and into the lump to be biopsied, while steadying a mobile lump with the fingers of the other hand.

4. Hold the needle still and advance the stylette further into the lump. Now hold the stylette still and advance the needle, which cuts off and encloses the tissue that bulged into the thinned section of the stylette. If the tissue is very hard, advance the closed needle into the lesion, hold the stylette still, withdraw then advance the needle to close it.
5. Draw out the closed needle, then retract the needle to expose the specimen resting on the thinned section of the stylette. Place the specimen in the appropriate fixative and immediately label the container, fill out the request form and ensure that the specimen is sent promptly to the laboratory.
6. A spring-loaded wide-bore needle can be used, or a drill biopsy – a high-speed rotating hollow needle.
7. All forms of needle biopsy may cause severe bleeding, so apply steady pressure over the track for 3–5 minutes, timed by the clock.

Open biopsy

Excision biopsy implies removing the whole structure or lesion such as a discrete lump on its own or lying within more homogeneous tissue. This is intended to remove the

lesion completely while providing material for histological examination. It is especially valuable if you think the lesion is, or could be, malignant; if this is a possibility, you wish to avoid transgressing into the lesion and potentially spreading tumour cells. In this case assiduously keep the plane of dissection in healthy tissue. Some lesions appear to have a capsule and the dissection may be extracapsular but the presence of a capsule does not preclude malignant penetration through it into the surrounding tissues.

> **Key points**
>
> - An apparent capsule may be merely compressed normal or abnormal tissues as a result of tumour expansion.
> - Even if there is a true capsule, it may have been infiltrated by malignant cells passing through to the surrounding tissues.

    Incision biopsy involves the removal of a portion from a large structure. It provides material for study but is not intended to remove the whole of the diseased tissue.

1. Always try to include junctional tissue between diseased and normal tissues, where the architecture is recognizable.
2. If an edge is present, excise a wedge from it, leaving a defect that can usually be closed with sutures (Fig. 7.3). If there is no edge, excise an ellipse in the shape of a boat with the keel lying in the depths (Fig. 7.4).
3. If you need to biopsy a deeply placed lump, make sure you can reach it safely without injuring nearby structures. You may have imaging views at 90° to each other as a guide. Be willing to make an adequate incision so you can identify structures you may encounter.
4. A *hooked wire marker* is used especially in the breast when a suspicious area such as a small mass or collection of microcalcification is identified on mammography or another imaging technique. As a rule the radiologist inserts a hollow needle into the suspicious area, introducing through this a hooked or curved wire before

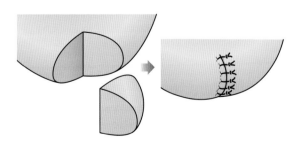

Fig. 7.3 Cut a wedge from the edge of a structure and appose the cut surfaces with stitches.

Fig. 7.4 Away from an edge, excise a boat-shaped specimen. If the tissue is supple you may be able to close the defect as a linear scar. If it is not, insert stitches and tie them, after drawing in nearby tissue to fill the defect, if possible. Alternatively, lay in gelatin foam or a similar haemostatic substance.

Fig. 7.5 The suspicious lesion has been identified by surface measurement, stereotactic measurement or ultrasound. After inserting a needle into it, pass through the needle a hooked or bent wire and then remove the needle. You may bend the wire and suture it flush with the skin to prevent it from being dislodged.

withdrawing the needle (Fig. 7.5). You should now approach the suspicious area by the most direct route. Cut through the outer part of the wire, leaving the hook marker in place. Excise the suspicious area and marker, if necessary taking X-rays of the specimen to confirm that the correct tissue has been excised.

CONNECTIVE TISSUE

This varies from flimsy areolar tissue, to tough ligaments, tendons and aponeuroses (G *apo* = from + *neuron* = nerve or tendon), which are flattened tendons attached to muscles. The vascularity of stable connective tissue is minimal but

blood vessels may cross connective tissue spaces, bound for other tissues and organs.

Tendons and aponeuroses have most of the fibres running in one direction – along the line of the attached muscle contraction.

Areolar tissue

Areolar tissue (L *areola*, diminutive of *area* = an open, empty place) occupies the space between structures that move relative to each other, for example between muscles, around tendons. It is an important guide to tissue planes and often has slack vessels crossing it to supply a moving structure such as a tendon or muscle, and from deep structures to supply mobile skin.

Cut it with scalpel or scissors, preferably after sealing any fine vessels with diathermy or harmonic scalpel. Occasionally it can be gently stripped with your fingers. Repair it using very fine absorbable stitches mounted on a round-bodied needle.

Aponeuroses

Because these transmit the pull of muscles the fibres tend to run parallel, although cross-fibres bind the parallel fibres together.

1. Whenever possible split them parallel to the fibres. If this is done they require minimal or no repair, since returning muscle tone pulls all the fibres straight, closing the constructed gap (see later, gridiron incision).
2. The cross-link fibres in aponeuroses that have been cut across the fibres are weak and single stitches may cut out. The tendency is reduced if you use horizontal mattress stitches (Fig. 7.6). For the same reason, when the fibres have been split and you repair it with sutures inserted at the same distance from the edge, they will separate off a strip if the aponeurosis is subjected to tension across the fibres. In this case insert the sutures at varying distances from the edges (Fig. 7.7). Healing of aponeuroses is slow. If they are subjected to strain at an early stage, the repair will give way or stretch. The ability to

Fig. 7.6 The aponeurosis has been cut across the fibres. **A** Simple stitches tend to cut out. **B** Horizontal mattress sutures hold better.

Fig. 7.7 The aponeurosis has been split between the fibres. **A** Stitches inserted all at the same distance from the edges tend to drag away a strip of fibres. **B** Stitches hold better if they are inserted at varying intervals from the edges.

stretch is increased during pregnancy, in nutritional deficiency and in old age. In some diseases there are molecular defects in collagen or elastic fibres.

3. Attempts to appose weak or stretched aponeuroses, especially if they are likely to come under tension, are usually doomed to failure. For many years surgeons attempted bridging of congenital and acquired parietal (L = a wall) defects. Sutures and darns inserted under tension swiftly or gradually give way. In the past biological and artificial materials were inserted, intended to create an inflammatory reaction, in the hope that fibrous tissue would be laid down. Non-absorbable synthetic meshes, usually of polypropylene or polyester, evoke little inflammatory reaction but are incorporated into the tissues. Cut a piece larger than the defect, so that it overlaps the edges, extending all round onto robust tissues without any tension, and suture or staple it in place (see later, hernia).

Key points

- Pulling edges of aponeurotic defects together with stitches has a high failure rate.
- Bridge the gap with tension-free plastic mesh.

Tendons

Tendons (G *teinein* = to stretch) are composed of aligned collagen and elastic fibres to transmit the pull of muscles. They have the highest tensile strength of any connective tissue. If they are split in the line of the fibres they often eventually heal without loss of strength. If they are transected across the fibres, the ends retract. Following repair the join is weak and stitches tend to cut out.

1. Stainless steel sutures were previously used but synthetic polyamide, polyester or polypropylene have improved the results. The larger the area of the repair the greater the chance of satisfactory union; consider cutting the ends obliquely or stepwise.
2. Tendon repairs are often performed after applying a tourniquet to ensure that the field is not obscured with blood.
3. Be particularly careful where a close-fitting tendon changes direction over a fibro-osseous pulley-like smooth ridge or under an aponeurotic band to prevent bow-stringing of the tendon, encased in a synovial sheath to reduce the friction. Do not injure the fine, mesentery-like connections (vinculae) bringing the blood supply from the deep surface, or the delicate mesothelial cells lining the synovium. If you leave an irregularity at such sites, adhesions develop between the tendon and the sheath, limiting or preventing movement.
4. If two tendons lying together have been divided, there is a danger that following repair of them both, they will adhere to each other or abrade each other. To prevent this, one of the tendons may be sacrificed. When the flexor digitorum profundus and superficialis of a finger are both divided, the superficialis tendon is usually not repaired.
5. Do not grasp the tendon ends with forceps; this will have a crushing effect, damaging and roughening the surface. Manipulate them with needles. One method is to transfix each of them with a straight needle about 2–2.5 cm from the cut ends. The needles can be drawn together and rotated as necessary to align the ends, but protect the needle points to prevent needle-stick injury. Make sure that the clean-cut ends come together, if necessary by flexing the join across which the tendon acts. The ends should fit together, without any twist, angulation or step.
6. Repair the tendon with a mattress stitch. Insert a stitch, usually of braided, synthetic polyester, into one end, emerging 1.5 cm from the end. Now reinsert the needle close to where it emerged, to cross the diameter of the tendon transversely, immediately opposite the point of insertion. Reinsert the needle close to the point of emergence, to reappear at the cut end. Bridge the gap between the cut ends and enter the other end, emerging 1.5 cm from the end, crossing the diameter of the tendon, back to the cut end (Fig. 7.8). It is often convenient to employ a straight needle but hold it with a needle-holder. Draw the two ends together, ensuring they fit without twisting. Tie a perfect knot that will lie between the ends, holding the ends in perfect apposition, without bunching. Finally insert a fine, monofilament, circumferential stitch to draw into continuity the paratenon, producing the smoothest possible surface.

Fig. 7.8 Repair of a tendon. **A** Insert stitches bridging the tendons. Draw the ends together and tie a knot that will be buried between the apposed ends. **B** Insert very fine continuous stitches to repair the paratenon.

7. Following repair, reduce tension to a minimum, by immobilizing joints in a position that brings the muscle origin and insertion as close as possible. Collagen laid down during healing stretches if it is strained, so unless the muscle pull is restrained, the tendon will be lengthened and subsequently the muscle action will be restricted.

8. When a tendon ruptures as it joins the bone, unite the ends provided the distal stump has retained its blood supply. Otherwise unite the proximal end into the bone. This is usually achieved by resecting a patch of cortical bone and drawing the tendon into contact with the underlying cancellous bone using non-absorbable stitches inserted through the tendon and through holes drilled through the bone.

Ligaments

These are bands or sheets of fibrous tissue connecting bones, cartilages and other structures (L *ligare* = to bind or tie), or act as supports for fascia, joints or muscles.

1. Torn supporting ligaments can often be repaired in a similar manner to aponeuroses or tendons.

2. Ligaments that stabilize joints such as collateral and cruciate ligaments of the knee are challenging to repair and demand specialist expertise. Unless they retain their length and strength, the joint becomes unstable. Some can be repaired like tendons. Cruciate ligaments of the knee can be repaired using either the tendons of hamstrings or the central portion of the patellar tendon with a piece of the tibia and the patella at each end, which can be anchored in tunnels within the femur and tibia. Allografts (G *allos* = other) such as bovine collateral ligament have been used, as well as a number of artificial materials such as carbon fibre, polyester and polytetrafluoroethylene.

NERVES

Nerve fibres are enclosed within, and protected by, the endoneurium; the perineurium encloses bundles or fasciculi of nerve fibres, and around the whole nerve is the epineurium (Fig. 7.9).

Neurapraxia (G *a* = not + *prassein* = to do) is a temporary physiological block.

Axonotmesis (G *temnein* = to cut) results from disruption of the axon but the endoneurium remains intact. Wallerian degeneration (Augustus Waller 1816–1870, English physiologist) occurs in the distal axon. The proximal axon sprouts distally along the intact endoneurial tube, eventually connecting with the end organ.

Neurotmesis results from division of the nerve. If the ends are coapted, axon sprouts enter the distal endoneurial tubes but the result is invariably less than perfect. Recovery of function is proportional to the perfection with which the original orientation is achieved so that axons enter the correct distal endoneurial tubes.

> **Key point**
>
> - The sooner you perform the repair and the more expertly you repair it, the better the result.

1. You may first need to eliminate infection and bleeding, achieve skeletal stability and assure primary skin closure. If you cannot fulfil these conditions, join the ends with a single stitch, close the skin or cover the nerve with well-vascularized tissue, elevate

Fig. 7.9 Repairing a cut nerve. Groups of fibres are encased in an endoneurial sheath (endoneurium), the fasciculi have a perineurium and the nerve has an epineurium. Ensure that the ends are brought into perfect alignment with the bundles correctly orientated, without tension or rotation. In some cases you need to use epineurial stitches only, in others you can connect the perineurial sheaths.

the part to prevent oedema and delay repair until the conditions are suitable.

2. Repair is usually carried out after applying a tourniquet to ensure there is adequate, bloodless exposure. Ensure that you have good light, available magnification with fine, microsurgical instruments and a loupe or operating microscope (see Ch. 5).
3. If the nerve ends are ragged, trim them with a razor blade so you can appose them in perfect orientation.
4. Carefully unite the epineurial sheaths using monofilament 8/0–10/0 nylon. In some cases fascicular repair is possible.
5. If a segment of the nerve is lost, or the ends have retracted, you may interpose a graft, usually taken from the sural (L *sura* = calf of the leg) nerve. This does, however, prejudice the final result. During parotidectomy for tumour, a branch of the facial nerve may be transacted or resected accidentally or deliberately because of tumour involvement. It is usual to bridge the gap with a segment of the great auricular nerve.
6. Following repair and closure in a limb, immobilize it in a position that avoids traction on the repair.

SKELETAL MUSCLE

Relaxed muscle is remarkably fragile and easily crushed. In contrast healthy contracted muscle is remarkably resistant to injury. If the motor nerve supply is lost the muscle is paralysed and atrophies (G *a* = not + *trephein* = to feed). If a muscle is transected, the muscle fibres do not reunite but they are connected by intervening fibrosis. The single muscle becomes double-bellied at best but the ends frequently distract, become attached to the muscle sheath and so lose their contractility.

It is a remarkable phenomenon for which I have never seen an explanation, that haematogenous metastases of neoplasms are rarely seen in skeletal muscle.

1. Apart from operating on muscles for local trauma or disease you frequently need to pass between or through them to reach your deeper surgical target. The muscles are often layered. Respect the fine external investing fascia which allows them to glide over each other without friction. The nerves and vessels usually enter from the deep surface (an exception is the serratus anterior muscle). Excessive displacement may prejudice the nerve and blood supply.
2. Re-appose muscle fibres running parallel to each other, and separated, using absorbable sutures mounted on round-bodied needles, but do not tie the sutures tightly or they will strangulate the muscle fibres and cut out. Indeed, in many situations it is unnecessary to insert sutures since once muscle tone returns, the fibres realign. Horizontal mattress stitches inserted to re-appose the ends of transacted muscles tend to cut out.

3. *Volkmann's ischaemic contracture*, described in 1872 by Richard Volkmann of Halle in Germany, results from muscle ischaemia. This can be caused by too tight encircling plaster, from swelling of muscle within inelastic fascia as in the anterior compartment of the lower leg, or pressure on, for example, the brachial artery following supracondylar fracture of the humerus. A too tight plaster can be split, a supracondylar fracture can be manipulated to relieve pressure on the artery. If the ischaemia is not relieved the muscle atrophies and is replaced with fibrous tissue; as this matures it shortens, causing contractures.
4. Encircling full-thickness burns of a limb have a similar effect to a tight plaster and usually the skin and often the deep fascia may need to be fully split longitudinally; such burns of the upper trunk cause restricted respiratory movement. They both demand immediate release by longitudinally splitting the eschar – the dry hard scab-like burned skin. This is the original meaning of debridement (F *débrider* = unbridle, release).
5. *Compartment syndrome* for example in the anterior compartment of the leg, from swelling of the muscle within the inelastic fascia, causes severe pain. If the pressure rises above 30 mmHg or differs less than 30 mmHg from diastolic pressure, severe necrosis is likely. It can be relieved by slitting the fascia and skin (open fasciotomy) to allow the muscle to bulge through. In some cases, this can be carried out subcutaneously if the fascia alone is causing the compression and the overlying skin is sufficiently slack. Compartment syndrome occurs elsewhere in the body and when the intra-abdominal contents swell, respiration and circulation are prejudiced and must be relieved.

CARTILAGE

1. Pure cartilage covers the ends of bones in contact at joints, or as menisci are interposed between bone ends. It has limited ability to regenerate because it has no intrinsic blood supply, usually obtaining it through the peripheral attachments. It usually heals with deposition of fibrocartilage.
2. Fibrocartilage can be cut and sutured and stitched after drilling stitch holes, and transplanted from one site to another as part of a composite graft.
3. The management of cartilaginous defects is in a state of flux as efforts are made to repair, renovate and regenerate it. Tears and dislocations that were formerly treated through open approaches, often involving total removal of intra-articular menisci of joints such as the knee, can now be repaired and smoothed using arthroscopic techniques.

MUCOPERIOSTEUM

This is a strong conjoint double layer with a good blood supply, covering among other areas the hard palate and bony nasal walls. It can be elevated from the bone as a flap to cover bony defects to close palatal defects in congenital cleft palate.

1. Choose the suture material depending on the feasibility of removing them. If they can be removed, use 3/0 black silk which is easy to see, or monofilament nylon which evokes minimal reaction, mounted on half-curved, reverse cutting, eyeless needles.
2. If it is difficult or impossible to remove stitches, insert 4/0 synthetic absorbable stitches.

BREAST

Breasts are glandular skin derivatives and supernumer-ary breasts may develop anywhere along the 'milk line' extending from the axilla to the groin. The consistency varies depending on the proportions of glandular and adipose tissue. The upper, outer quadrant and axillary tail tend to have denser glandular tissue than elsewhere. This variation makes it difficult to differentiate lumpiness from lump.

1. Cysts can be aspirated and the fluid sent for cytological examination. Deeply placed cysts may be reached guided by ultrasound imaging.
2. During lactation retained milk may produce galactoceles (G *galaktos* = milk + *kele* = a swelling) and infection of the breast can result in cellulitis and abscess formation. At an early stage antibiotics may thwart abscess formation but if an abscess forms, the pus can often be aspirated as an alternative to open drainage.
3. Palpable lumps can be investigated with fine-needle aspiration cytology (FNAC) or needle biopsy.
4. Impalpable doubtful lumps detected by imaging can be marked with a hooked wire if open biopsy needs to be carried out.
5. *Open biopsy* is occasionally required when the diagnosis is in doubt. Carry out excision biopsy unless the lump is very large, in which case remove a thin slice for histological examination. Place the incision so that it can be incorporated within a wider incision if this proves necessary. Avoid damaging the architecture. Hold on to attached connective tissue, not the lump itself. Do not try to close the gap but obtain perfect haemostasis before carefully closing the skin.

6. When operating on the breast constantly bear in mind the radial distribution of the lobules which drain centrally to reach the nipple. Plan incisions to take into account the cosmetic result. Skin tension lines are mainly transverse before the breast develops but as it fills and eventually sags they change.
7. Avoid the development of a haematoma by achieving perfect haemostasis.
8. For localized carcinoma employ a wider excision, keeping well clear of the lump. As a safeguard against local recurrence the cavity walls may be resected when the lump has been removed.
9. A more certain procedure is *quadrantectomy*, removing a quarter of the breast down to the pectoral muscles like a quarter of a round cake, from nipple to periphery. It may be combined with limited or complete axillary lymph node clearance or sentinel node biopsy (see below). Do not attempt to close the gap in the breast. Close the skin after attaining perfect haemostasis.
10. *Modified radical mastectomy* is the total removal of the whole breast including the axillary tail down to the chest wall but preserving the pectoral muscles and chest wall, and including clearance of the axillary glands, described by David Patey of the Middlesex Hospital London in 1948. It is a modification of the operation devised by William Halsted of Baltimore (1852–1922), which included resecting the pectoral muscles.

LYMPH NODES

Enlargement of lymph nodes indicates local inflamma-tion, infection, malignant or other disease; alternatively it may be a local manifestation of generalized disease.

Enlarged nodes may be singular, multiple, discrete, mat-ted, mobile or fixed. Superficial enlarged nodes are usually palpable although the physical signs may be misleading. Infected subfascial nodes may rupture, forming an abscess which may then burst through the fascia to present subcu-taneously; this is a 'collar-stud' abscess.

Deeply placed nodes can be demonstrated by various methods of imaging, or displayed at operation.

1. Before operation discuss with the pathologist how to prepare the specimen, and which receptacles are needed.
2. Carry out fine-needle aspiration cytology and needle biopsy only if you are confident of the anatomy, otherwise recruit the aid of a radiologist who can use ultrasound or other imaging methods for guidance.
3. Lymph nodes are fragile and if they are crushed the accuracy of the diagnosis is prejudiced.

Key points

- Lymph node biopsy is not a minor or casual procedure; most nodes are in close proximity to important structures.
- Never attempt to remove a node without studying the anatomy and obtaining adequate exposure. Many surgical disasters result from a cavalier attitude to removing what appears to be a solitary, mobile lymph node.

4. Place the incision in a skin crease if possible and approach the node with caution. Lymph nodes may be very fragile, especially if they are diseased. Having reached the surface of the node, work around the sides but do not grasp it with forceps because you may damage it; if possible leave a little connective tissue attached to it so that you can grasp this.
5. As you reach the deeper aspects, move the mobilized gland from side to side so that you can examine its attachments from different aspects. Remember that the vessels usually enter from the undersurface and that there may be an adherent important structure. The majority of complications arise because we are tempted to lift the gland, put the resulting pedicle under tension, cut it – and often regret it.
6. Carefully check the field and ensure total haemostasis.
7. On occasion you must remove one or a few glands from a matted mass of glands. Do not damage glands you do not intend to remove.
8. Divide up the node, without crushing it, into the required number of specimens and place them in the appropriate receptacles.
9. Close the wound to give the best possible cosmetic result.

Sentinel node biopsy

1. Before operation for diagnosed breast carcinoma, a peritumoral injection of a radioactive substance such as ^{99m}Tc-labelled nanocolloid may be injected around the tumour.
2. It is taken up by lymphatics and carried to the lymph nodes where it can be detected using a gamma probe. This first draining node can be removed and examined to detect cancer cells. Alternatively or as well, vital blue dye can be injected around the tumour and seen to track within the lymphatics to the glands (Fig. 7.10). If the removed gland is free of tumour cells it is unlikely, though still possible, that the cancer has spread more widely in the lymphatic system.
3. The technique may be used to determine the extent of spread of other neoplasms such as malignant melanoma (Ch. 6) and oesophageal adenocarcinoma.

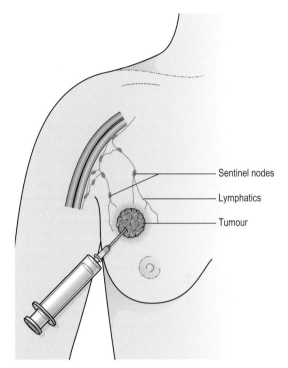

Fig. 7.10 Sentinel node biopsy as an aid to determine the extent of breast cancer dissemination and so decide the extent of the resection. A radioactive substance is injected around the tumour and tracked to the sentinel nodes using a gamma probe. Alternatively or in addition, vital blue dye may be injected and identified in the lymphatics passing to the glands. Histology of the excised glands offer guidance on the extent of tumour spread.

ABDOMINAL WALL

The usual purpose of incisions in the abdomen is to achieve the best possible access to structures within the cavity. The descriptions are intended merely to outline the steps of the frequently performed procedures. Whenever possible, avoid cutting through muscle. This can be achieved in two standard incisions, a midline vertical and a 'gridiron' incision for appendicectomy.

Midline abdominal incision

1. As a rule you stand on the supine patient's right side.
2. The incision divides the skin, linea alba and peritoneum in the upper or lower abdomen, or central abdomen by skirting the umbilicus. Divide the skin with the belly of the scalpel, holding the knife so that it cuts vertically without slicing. Start at the upper end, cutting from your left to right.
3. After achieving haemostasis, continue in the same line through the white, firm, fibrous linea alba and

then stop as you reach a variable layer of fat overlying the fused fascia transversalis and peritoneum.

4. Pick up the final layer with the tips of a haemostat to tent it, allowing you to grasp it again, alongside the first grip. Remove and then replace the first forceps while holding up the peritoneum with the second forceps, to allow any viscus inadvertently picked up by the first forceps to slip clear. Now have both haemostats held up, tenting the peritoneum while you make a small incision between them. This allows air to enter the abdomen so that viscera can fall clear (Fig. 7.11). Insert a finger into the peritoneal cavity and move it in a complete circle to confirm that there is no viscus in danger. Having assured yourself, insert one blade of Mayo's scissors and carefully slit the peritoneum in the line of the initial incision.

5. To close the incision, grasp the peritoneum at each end with strong, straight haemostatic forceps and have them lifted clear of the underlying viscera by your assistant. You may also apply similar forceps in the middle of each edge, allowing the handles to lie outwards, everting the edges. Insert a non-absorbable suture such as 1 monofilament nylon mounted on a round-bodied curved needle. Alternatively, the sutures can be mounted on blunt taper-point needles that will penetrate the tissues but do not easily penetrate surgical gloves or the skin. Absorbable synthetic sutures are popular with many surgeons because their strength is reliably retained for a period before they are absorbed.

6. It is usually most convenient to suture from the upper end to the lower, from your non-dominant to your dominant side, as the incision lies transversely in front of you. Take a bite through all layers, except the skin and subcutaneous tissues, from out to in on the far side, in to out on the near side, and tie the suture securely. Ensure that the bristly short end is well buried. Alternatively you may use a thinner suture that has both ends inserted into the needle, forming a closed loop. Insert your first stitch, then pass the needle through the loop – this produces a less bulky means of securing the start of the suture line.

7. Insert a continuous, over-and-over stitch until you reach the other end. Drive the needle from without in on the far side, from within out on the near side, approximately every 1 cm, placed 1 cm from the edge, forming a spiral within the tissues. This allows the stitches to adjust so that the tension is equalized between them.

8. Carefully avoid over-tightening the stitches. Once you have apposed the edges, have your assistant steady the emerging thread so you can avoid the sawing action of tightening, slackening and retightening the stitches.

9. Take care to avoid injuring structures with the last few stitches by inserting them slackly, with the edges separated, then tightening them seriatim.

10. At the end, hold on to the final loop on one side and the single thread on the other. You may either tie the loop to the single thread or employ an Aberdeen knot (see Ch. 3).

11. As a rule do not insert subcutaneous stitches.

12. Now carefully close the skin with interrupted or continuous stitches.

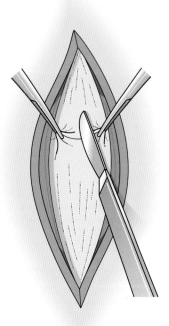

Fig. 7.11 Incising the peritoneum after tenting it between two forceps.

Key points

- Ceaselessly and vigilantly protect the abdominal contents from injury.
- Place every stitch carefully, through all the intended layers.
- Do not damage the suture material or you will weaken it.
- Over-tightened stitches strangle the tissues and are likely to cut out, risking burst abdomen.
- Tie knots securely and turn the bristly ends under, so they do not project under the skin.

Gridiron incision

1. The incision is named after the crossed iron bars laid over a fire on which to grill food, resembling the crossed lateral abdominal muscle layers. It is associated with the New York surgeon Charles McBurney (1845–1913), who established the diagnosis and surgical treatment of appendicitis. He described a point in the right iliac fossa at the junction of the middle and outer thirds of a line between the umbilicus and anterior superior iliac spine where the maximal tenderness is felt in the disease and on which the incision is centred.

2. Make the skin incision centred on the point. McBurney's skin incision was at right angles to the spino-umbilical line with one third above, two thirds below his point. Otto Lanz of Amsterdam (1865–1935) described an incision along the skin crease which results in a more cosmetically acceptable scar. Incise the subcutaneous tissue in the same line.

3. You expose the shining aponeurosis of external oblique muscle. Split the fibres without cutting them, to reveal the fibres of internal oblique muscle, at right angles to the external oblique. Split these to reveal the fibres of transversus abdominis muscle. For each layer, make a small incision with a scalpel, then gently insert the tips of Mayo's scissors into the gap and open them in the line of the fibres. Split these to reveal the conjoint transversalis fascia and peritoneum (Fig. 7.12).

4. Pick up the peritoneum with artery forceps to tent it, grasp the raised tented portion, release and re-grasp the peritoneum with the first forceps. Have the two forceps held up while you make a small scalpel incision between them, to let in air and allow the viscera to fall away. Insert a finger to ensure that there is no adherent structure before introducing one blade of a pair of scissors to enlarge the opening fully within the muscle boundaries.

5. Close the incision in layers. First hold up the ends of the peritoneal incision and insert a continuous suture of 2/0 or 3/0 absorbable synthetic suture to close it, ensuring you do not injure any intra-abdominal structure. Using the same material, insert interrupted stitches to appose each of the muscle layers, taking care not to pull the stitches tight. Finally close the skin using interrupted or continuous sutures. To achieve a good cosmetic result you may wish to insert a subcuticular stitch (see Ch. 6).

Hernia

Defects in aponeuroses congenitally acquired or from trauma, atrophy or paralysis may allow deep structures to

Fig. 7.12 The gridiron incision for appendicectomy. Split but do not cut the fibres of the aponeurosis and muscles to reach the peritoneum.

bulge. Such a protrusion is a hernia. Plastic mesh repair has transformed the repair, notably in the groin and following incisional hernias following failed repairs of abdominal incisions.

1. Expose the superficial layer of the bulge, which is the peritoneum in abdominal hernias, and define the margins of the defect. You may be able to invaginate the bulge.

2. If the hernia bulges into an elongated sac you must first reduce the contents, if necessary after opening the sac, then close the neck of the sac and excise the excess.

3. Lay the mesh, with generous overlap of the defect edges, superficial to the defect, or under the deep surface from within the underlying cavity.

4. Fix the mesh using simple sutures or staples (Fig. 7.13).

5. An abdominal wall hernia may be repaired transperitoneally using laparoscopic methods from within the abdominal cavity. Alternatively it can be approached extraperitoneally after creating a space between the abdominal wall and peritoneum, then expanding it with an inflatable balloon.

6. This tension-free technique is highly successful. The mesh is well tolerated. Fibroblasts lay down collagen fibres that embed it securely in the tissues.

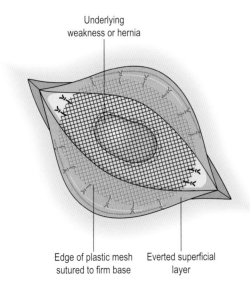

Underlying
weakness or hernia

Edge of plastic mesh   Everted superficial
sutured to firm base   layer

Fig. 7.13 Plastic mesh tension-free repair of a hernia. The superficial tissues have been undermined and the mesh laid in, generously overlapping the margins. It is now sutured or stapled in place and then covered over and the wound is closed.

ABDOMINAL CONTENTS

Bowel

Provided the normally rich blood supply is intact and edges are carefully apposed, bowel (L *botellus* = a sausage) heals well (see Ch. 4). Although the contents of the small bowel are normally almost sterile, as soon as there is any stagnation, microorganisms flourish here, as they normally do in the colon.

> **Key point**
>
> • Repaired bowel must have: a good blood supply, perfect apposition of the edges, absence of tension.

Liver

1. Liver is honeycombed with blood vessels and bile ducts so that it bleeds and oozes bile when cut. The capsule, described by Francis Glisson of Bristol about 1677, encloses the liver, extending into the porta hepatis, and is of variable strength.
2. Liver is amenable to fine-needle aspiration or to needle biopsy. Ultrasound or other imaging methods may be used to guide the needle to lesions. A long, fine 'skinny' needle can be inserted percutaneously into the intrahepatic bile ducts and contrast media injected into them to produce a cholangiogram (G *chole* = bile

+ *angeion* = vessel + *graphein* = to write). By using the Seldinger technique (see Ch. 5), the biliary system can be entered, and a guidewire passed through the common bile duct and into the duodenum. Following the passage of dilators over the guidewire, stents can be placed across a stenotic section.

3. In the presence of bleeding oesophageal varices secondary to cirrhosis and portal venous hypertension, a number of procedures can be performed. The anastomotic channels draining the hypertensive portal venous system into the systemically drained oesophageal veins can be disconnected, or the portal vein can be drained directly into the inferior vena cava – portacaval shunt. This can now be achieved percutaneously by creating a transhepatic intrajugular portal-systemic shunt (TIPS) within the liver. A guidewire is passed down the right internal jugular vein, superior vena cava, right atrium, inferior vena cava, right hepatic vein, then through liver substance and via a tributary, into the portal vein. A stent is placed across as a bridge, creating a portal/systemic conduit.
4. At operations on the liver, bleeding and bile leakage can be controlled using diathermy current and employing blunt dissection. 'Finger fracture' consists of compressing a portion of liver between finger and thumb, crushing the liver cells but not dividing the vessels and ducts; these can then be identified, doubly ligated and divided. Ultrasound, electrosurgical, high-pressure water jet, laser, and radiofrequency methods are used to facilitate liver resection without causing excessive blood loss (see Ch. 9). Oozing surfaces can be sealed using a variety of applied haemostatic materials, and an argon beam can be used to carry an electrosurgical high-frequency current to the surface, coagulating the vessels with minimal penetration.
5. After achieving haemostasis, absorbable synthetic sutures mounted on large round-bodied curved needles can be inserted to appose the cut surfaces. Take bites well away from the cut edges and tighten them only just sufficient to appose the surfaces or they will cut out. In some cases it is beneficial to insert stitches parallel with the edges to slightly constrict and support them before placing stitches to appose the cut edges (Fig. 7.14).

Spleen

In the past splenectomy was carried out with little concern, as part of other procedures, even if it was only slightly damaged. This aggressive attitude stemmed from the propensity of the damaged spleen to continue to bleed or develop recurrent bleeding.

The dangers of post-splenectomy infection are now recognized, especially in children, so that it is preserved whenever possible.

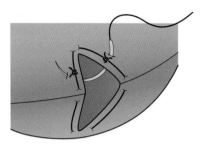

Fig. 7.14 Suture the liver using a large, round-bodied needle. It may be an advantage to insert an encircling stitch close to the edges before bringing the edges together with apposing stitches placed outside these.

1. A capsular tear may seal if you apply haemostatic agents such as fibrin glue, gelatin sponge, polyglycolic mesh, microfibrillar collagen or crushed muscle.
2. If there is a tear into the pulp, consider inserting stitches to close it, if necessary tying the stitches over gelatin sponge or a tongue of omentum.
3. If you need to remove the spleen, consider placing slices of the spleen into pockets constructed in the greater omentum.
4. Determine to give anti-pneumococcal vaccine postoperatively. Advise adults to seek treatment at the first sign of infection and give children prophylactic penicillin for 2 years.

Pancreas

The pancreas (G *pas* = all + *kreas* = flesh) is well protected from injury but is very fragile. If the enzymes are released and activated they are extremely erosive.
1. The gland does not hold stitches well, so repair is difficult to achieve.
2. The body or the tail can be removed, followed by closure of the main duct.
3. Close the parenchyma. This may be conveniently achieved by cutting the stump in the shape of a fishtail (Fig. 7.15), and suturing the edges.

UROLOGICAL SYSTEM

Kidney

This has a rich blood supply, a firm capsule which holds stitches well and it is amenable to repair provided the

Fig. 7.15 Repairing the pancreas. Cut the stump end like a fish tail and suture together the two flaps you have created.

drainage system is intact. The vessels are end arteries so partial nephrectomy must reflect the distribution. Control the bleeding, insert fine absorbable sutures to close collecting system defects and insert absorbable stitches through the capsule, crossing the parenchyma tied just tightly enough to appose the tissues without them cutting out.

Ureter

This must be sutured with fine stitches to avoid obstructing the narrow channel (see Ch. 4). If it must be repaired in the lower part, it may be preferable to join it directly to the bladder by raising a flap of bladder roof formed into a tube to bridge the gap, described by Boari in 1894.

Bladder

The wall is robust and holds sutures well. Many urologists exclude the lining epithelium from the stitches, which catch all the other layers.

Testis

Torsion of the testis is treated whenever possible by untwisting it and fixing it, and its twin, to the scrotum to prevent recurrence. Whenever possible, undescended testis is freed and brought down into the scrotum. For the treatment of malignant disease the testis is removed with ligation of the vas deferens and blood vessels.

In order to perform male sterilization the spermatic cord is identified and under local anaesthesia, incised to expose the vas deferens. A section is excised, both ends closed and the upper end is buried to avoid the possibility of reconnection.

Penis

Apart from cultural reasons *circumcision* needs to be performed only for phimosis (G = muzzling). It needs to be performed expertly. As a rule the foreskin is first incised dorsally to enable the adhesions between it and the glans to be gently separated. The prepuce is excised circumferentially while preserving the frenulum (Latin *frenum* = bridle) on the undersurface. After achieving perfect haemostasis, the two layers are joined together with interrupted, fine, absorbable sutures.

GYNAECOLOGICAL SYSTEM

Uterus

The thick muscle is tough and holds stitches well, following for example, caesarean section to deliver a child when vaginal delivery fails or sometimes for other reasons. However, the suture line leaves a scar that is relatively weak compared with the remainder of the wall. The uterine tubes have a narrow lumen. If they are to be repaired, use the finest sutures inserted with great care, preferably with magnification (see Ch. 4). Fibroids can usually be dissected free. Very large ones can sometimes be reduced in size by thermo-ablation or diathermy. Hysterectomy (G *hystera* = womb) may be necessary for large, multiple fibroids or uterine cancer.

Ovaries

Formerly the only common procedure carried out on the ovaries was removal but whenever possible they are treated by conservative surgery and also they may in part or whole be preserved by freezing.

CARDIORESPIRATORY SYSTEM

Lung

The lung remains expanded because it fills the intermittently sub-atmospheric pleural cavity. It collapses if air enters the potential space through either a breach in the chest wall or a damaged lung.

1. A leak usually reseals if you insert a chest drain connected to an underwater seal (see Ch. 11).
2. Suture large tears in the lung using absorbable synthetic sutures.
3. Each area is supplied with arteries, veins and bronchi allowing resection of a lung, lobe or segment.

Heart

Heart muscle holds stitches well and they can be inserted while the heart continues to beat. It is possible to stop the heart and bypass its pump action in order to perform delicate procedures on it such as valve replacement within the lumen. Pericardiocentesis should now be performed with the aid of two-dimensional echocardiography to avoid complications.

ENDOCRINE SYSTEM

Glandular tissue is relatively soft but the connective tissue usually provides good support. The thyroid gland is vascular, especially in thyrotoxic states. Surgery of the thyroid gland demands intimate knowledge of the anatomy. At risk are major blood vessels, the recurrent laryngeal nerves and the parathyroid glands. (See also Ch. 8, Tissue planes, p. 155.) The adrenal gland is fragile and has small veins that are easily torn. It is now usually operated upon by minimal access techniques.

BRAIN AND SPINAL CORD

These are extremely fragile. If they are damaged, healing is by the deposition of connective glial (G = glue) tissue. The unmyelinated nerve fibres cannot reunite, although the brain is 'plastic', in that it appears to be able to use alternative connections in response to lost tracts.

A further difficulty with some tumours is in differentiating them from normal brain. Modern imaging aids such as computerized tomography (CT) display brain abnormalities including displacements. Magnetic resonance imaging following intravenous gadolinium-DPTA highlights tumour vascularity and is valuable in outlining the margins of tumours.

1. Nerve tracts can be approached within the brain and in the spinal cord by direct approach or by stereotactic (G *stereos* = solid, three-dimensional + *tassein* = to arrange) techniques.
2. The brain is richly supplied with blood vessels which may become blocked or bleed. These may be treatable by interventional radiographic techniques. Extradural vessels such as the middle meningeal vessels may bleed following a cranial fracture, lifting the periosteum and dura, reducing the intracranial space. Sudden impacts or rotations may tear the veins crossing from the brain to the intracranial venous sinuses, resulting in subdural haemorrhage. Aneurysms in the circle of Willis may rupture, causing subarachnoid haemorrhage. Vessels within the brain may rupture, causing intracerebral bleeding, or they may clot – intracerebral thrombosis producing a 'stroke'. Narrowed vessels may give rise to transient ischaemic attacks (TIAs).
3. Operations on the brain present special difficulties because in most areas the brain tissue of obvious functional areas and what were in the past considered 'silent' areas, do not differ in appearance. The cortex was mapped by surgeons, such as Wilder Penfield 1891–1976 in Montreal, using an electrical probe while operating under local anaesthesia on conscious patients. In order to detect incipient functional damage when operating close to vital areas, neurosurgeons often carry out intracranial operations with the patient conscious and monitored.
4. Advanced three-dimensional imaging methods allow tumours to be accurately located. As an alternative to open surgery, many can be treated in a single session using Gamma Knife irradiation. Multiple, narrow intersecting beams are focused on the tumour with minimal damage to the surrounding normal brain.

Chapter | 8 |

Handling bone and joints

Bone

PHYSICAL CHARACTERISTICS

1. Although it appears rigid and static, bone is complex, flexible and dynamic. Long bones must grow as a child develops towards adult size. At one or usually both the ends of the main central section, the diaphysis (G *dia* = between + *phyein* = to bring forth – to grow), is a growing bone, a hyaline cartilage growth plate – the physis, beyond which are the ends, the epiphyses (G *epi* = upon). The epiphyses commonly participate in joints. The part of the diaphysis beneath the physis continuing to grow until maturity is the metaphysis (G *meta* = apart). Make every effort to protect the growth plates – the perichondrial ring – from damage. Recognize and allow for this in growing children.

2. The architectural structure of a long bone is complex. The outer cortex is compact with a porosity of only 5–10%. Successive layers of collagen fibrils, orientated at right angles to each other like plywood, form an elastic matrix with great tensile (L *tendere* = to stretch) strength. On this are deposited crystals of calcium phosphate, providing rigidity and high compression strength but low tensile strength. The medulla is cancellous – a latticework, with a porosity of over 50%. The distribution is not haphazard – trabeculae (L small beams) carry the weight to the cortex, especially near joint surfaces.

3. Bone is absorbed or deposited in response to the imposed stresses of gravity and activity, probably mediated by a piezo-electric (G *piezein* = to press; electricity generated by strain on certain crystals)

effect and streaming potential changes in the bone fluids. The bone undergoes demineralization during inactivity but in the presence of continued high stress the compact cortex increases; osteoclasts first create space in which osteoblasts form mineralized tubular Haversian canals (John Havers, 1650–1702, London anatomist and physician). The bone surface is covered with periosteum, consisting of an outer durable connective tissue layer covering an inner cambium layer rich in osteoblasts; these form the primary source of cells uniting a fracture or osteotomy, so avoid crushing or unnecessary stripping. Be aware of and preserve the bone blood supply. Apart from the nutrient artery which pierces the diaphysis giving ascending and descending medullary arteries, vessels enter at muscle, tendon, ligament and capsular insertions, especially around the metaphysis.

4. Infection of bone tends to become chronic and responds poorly to antibiotics. During operations sedulously avoid contamination by adhering to a 'no touch' technique, using instruments rather than fingers to manipulate bone whenever possible, and wearing two pairs of gloves.

5. Bony union, following fracture or osteotomy, occurs only if the surfaces are brought into fairly close contact or if the gap is filled with bone graft. Perfect apposition, absence of movement and compression of the fragments achieves primary union. A haematoma develops if there is movement or separation of the fragments; this is invaded in turn by granulation tissue, cartilage and osteoid tissue, called 'callus', which later ossifies. Rigid fixation allows early return of function and weight-bearing, avoiding joint stiffness and muscle wasting. It is, though, recognized that a slight degree of movement encourages healing.

6. Take into account your patients' ages – biological age may be more important than calendar age – gender, nutritional status and any co-morbidity, since their reaction to operation and subsequent healing is markedly influenced by them.

EXPOSURE

1. Many approaches are standardized – learn and apply them to avoid damaging overlying structures. Equally important is avoidance of unnecessary periosteal stripping, and damage to the perichondrial ring around the physis in children.

2. This is no excuse for failing to revise the anatomy of the whole area because missiles, trauma and invasive diseases are not respecters of anatomical planes. You may need to explore beyond the intended limits.

Fig. 8.1 Use a self-retaining retractor and a bone lever to expose a long bone. Have your assistant steady the bone with bone-holding forceps.

Steadying

1. Do not work on unfixed and unsteadied bone with sharp, and especially powered sharp, tools. Your tools will inevitably slip and damage the bone and vital soft tissues.

2. Make use of retractors, levers, forceps, guard plates, swabs and your assistants to protect the tissues from inadvertent damage (Fig. 8.1).

3. If you change your point of attack, reassess your safeguards and if necessary rearrange them.

BIOPSY

1. Although imaging methods have developed, histological diagnosis may still be required to elucidate general and bone disease.

2. If the area is soft, diagnostic cells can be recovered using fine-needle aspiration cytology or Trucut® introduced percutaneously and guided by imaging methods if necessary.

3. Under local anaesthesia, through a small skin incision you may obtain a bone marrow specimen using a Jamishidi type needle – a hollow needle with a cutting edge. This is rotated in a reciprocal fashion to pierce the cortex. Larger amounts can be obtained by multiple punctures, especially from the posterior iliac crests. The needle is used in an emergency to infuse fluids into the bone marrow when venous access is difficult; suitable sites include the tibia one finger's breadth medial to the tuberosity, and the

humeral head. A circular trephine cuts by rotating it like a circular pastry cutter. Guided biopsy may be performed under imaging control.

4. Open biopsy, usually under general anaesthesia, requires exposure of the bone. Use cutting tools to remove bone; soft tissues can be removed with a knife or curette.

CUTTING

Hand saw

1. Hand saws are infrequently used now, even for major amputations.
2. Decide the line of the cut and expose it fully, clear of other structures.
3. Protect the soft tissues in the line of the cut and those that might be damaged if the saw blade slips. If you cover them you also protect them from bone dust.
4. Hand saws are designed to make straight cuts. Do not attempt to change the line of the cut or you risk jamming the blade. Start a fresh line.
5. First create a starter groove by drawing the blade towards you, while steadying it against your non-dominant thumb placed well above the teeth (Fig. 8.2).

Key point

- Remember that saws remove a wider thickness of bone than the thickness of the blade, because of the 'set' of the teeth.

6. In some cases you can use a saw guide.
7. Use a steady, rhythmic, to-and-fro movement, the full length of the blade, putting no downward pressure on the saw. The teeth cut as you push the saw away from you.

Fig. 8.2 Start the saw cut by drawing the blade towards you, steadying the blade with the non-dominant thumb placed high up on the blade.

8. At the end of the cut avoid putting a strain on the bone or you will fracture it. Prefer to lighten the movement so that the last section does not suddenly give way. In some cases you can make a counter-cut from the opposite side, so the break occurs away from the edge and avoids leaving a sharp projecting splinter.

Gigli saw

The cutting wire can be passed under a bone, or a portion of bone demarcated with access through holes. Attach handles at each end and draw the saw, using a reciprocal motion, towards the surface, sawing within the bone, thus reducing the risk of damaging deep structures (Fig. 8.3).

Powered saws (Fig. 8.4)

1. Power is by electricity or compressed air. Circular rotation is potentially dangerous because the unengaged portion of the blade is liable to damage other tissues – or you. A reciprocating (L *re* = backwards + *pro* = forwards) saw is less dangerous.
2. Radially oscillating (L *oscillare* = to swing) blades, sawing in a small segment of arc only, at approximately 15 000 cycles/second, reduce the cutting areas.
3. High-speed saws produce a fine cloud of bone particles. Protect surrounding tissues or they will be covered with bone swarf, which is a potential contaminant.

Fig. 8.3 The Gigli wire saw can be passed under the bone, handles attached and drawn on in turn, to cut up to the surface.

135

Fig. 8.4 Powered saws are of two types. **A** A reciprocating saw moves the blade back and forth in the same manner as a hand saw (see Fig. 8.2). **B** A powered oscillating saw blade moves in a limited segment of a circle.

4. The saw blade heats up during long cuts, overheating bone in contact with it, which will die. Continually cool the blade with sterile saline solution.
5. Do not use blunt blades in powered saws – they cut unreliably.

Key points

- Protect the tissues from inadvertent damage and bone swarf.
- Wear eye protection to avoid getting 'splatter' into your own eyes.
- Avoid overheating bone or it will subsequently die. Use saline irrigation.
- Be doubly careful when nearing the end of the cut in case the saw rapidly over-runs the desired course.

Fig. 8.6 Cutting with an osteotome or chisel. Steady the hand holding the tool to prevent it from slipping to one side or cutting right through the bone and damaging soft tissues beyond.

Osteotome

1. This is thin, has bevels on both sides and is designed to make only straight cuts (Fig. 8.5A) rather than destroy bone, as opposed to a chisel which has a bevel on one side.

2. Plan the cut carefully to avoid deviation, which would strain the thin metal shaft.
3. Hold the osteotome in your non-dominant hand and drive it using a short-handed mallet to limit the striking force (Fig. 8.6).
4. To prevent shattering the sometimes brittle cortical bone, either first drill holes in the line of the cut or first cut chips out of the cortex so it can accommodate the thickness of the blade (Fig. 8.7).

Key point

- Steady the hand, holding the osteotome in such a way that you prevent the tool from slipping to one side or cutting through the bone into the soft tissues beyond.

Fig. 8.5 **A** Osteotome. **B** Chisel. **C** Gouge.

Chisel

1. The bevel (Fig. 8.5B) on the chisel (OF *cisel* from L *caedere* = to cut), also driven by a short-handled mallet, resists cutting along a straight path.
2. If you place the chisel on a bony surface, bevel uppermost and tap it, it may chip off a flake of

Fig. 8.7 Widen the cut as the osteotome bites deeper by successively chipping flakes from each side so that the thickness of the instrument can be accommodated to prevent splitting.

superficial bone (Fig. 8.8). As it bites, the bevel makes it angle deeper so that the handle swings more vertically. There is danger that because of the thickness of the chisel, it will fracture the bone.

3. If the bevel is on the undersurface, you need to start the cut with the tool held more vertically or it will fail to bite, and will slide along the surface. As soon as the bevel enters the bone, the chisel tends to lift the edge on the unbevelled side and the handle is angled downwards. When you drive the chisel further, the effect of the bevel is to guide the cutting edge towards the surface, lifting off a sliver (OE *slifan* = to cleave) of superficial bone, as the chisel lies almost parallel with the surface.
4. A gouge (Fig.8.5C), has a hollow blade to scoop out. The bevel is on the outside so that it does not bite deeply. It is useful for harvesting cancellous bone.

Cutting forceps

1. These act like scissors (Fig. 8.9) so that you can make small cuts through bone that is not too thick or brittle, such as a rib, although a special guillotine type of tool is available for this purpose.
2. It inevitably has a crushing effect on the bone. In case of doubt, therefore, prefer to use a saw when this is appropriate.

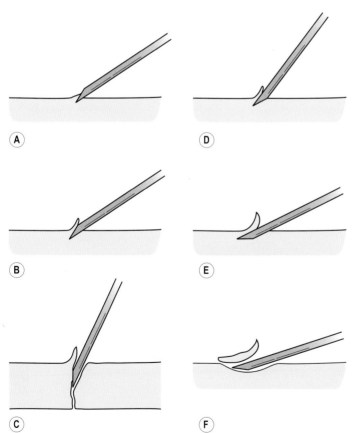

Fig. 8.8 Driving a chisel into bone. **A** Bevel uppermost. **B** It tends to angle vertically as it bites more deeply. **C** It becomes even more vertical and may split the bone. **D** Bevel on the underside. **E** The chisel tip lifts a sliver of bone and tends to flatten. **F** The chisel has cut out and lies almost parallel with the bone surface.

Fig. 8.9 Bone cutting forceps at top. Rongeurs at centre and bottom; these have cupped blades so fragments of detached bone are grasped but not crushed, and can be removed.

Rongeurs

1. There are several versions of these (Fig. 8.9) and as the name implies (F *ronger* = to gnaw), they nibble away bone, especially in difficult corners or cavities.
2. They are valuable where a power tool or an osteotome may endanger vital tissues as in spinal laminectomy.
3. Rongeurs are useful for obtaining specimens for histology from bone or other hard tissues. Because the jaws are hollowed out, they do not excessively crush and destroy the architecture of the specimens.

File

Because bone is not homogeneous like metal and wood, files tend to be used only for rasping sharp edges from angular cuts made with saws and other instruments, as following an amputation.

Fig. 8.11 Brace and tools for opening the skull. At the top is a perforator and below are two types of burrs.

DRILLING

1. Hand drills (Fig 8.10) are not now used routinely for drilling bone. It may be difficult to start the hole, especially on rounded, hard, cortical bone, without first making a preliminary notch with an awl or sharp punch, otherwise the drill point tends to 'walk' away from the intended point of penetration.
2. Because both hands are fully occupied with holding and turning the drill it is difficult to control. Limit the penetration of the cutting bit by ensuring that only the required length protrudes from the chuck, or fix a clamp to the bit which acts as a buffer when it hits the bone surface.
3. A hand brace (Fig. 8.11), can be used as when trephining the skull; in this case the bit is not a drill but a shaped cutting perforator that prevents sudden uncontrolled penetration. The opening in the skull can then be enlarged using burrs, which act like circular rasps.
4. Powered drills (Fig. 8.12), are now routinely employed. Properly controlled, they allow you to concentrate on the process of drilling without the need to turn the bit yourself. Since they rotate at a higher speed than manual drills, they may easily 'run away'. Identify and carefully protect vulnerable soft tissues from damage and from the spray of bone dust.

Fig. 8.10 Hand drill.

Fig. 8.12 Powered drill.

Fig. 8.13 Drill guides. The one on the left is hand-held; the one on the right can be firmly attached to the bone, leaving you two hands to control the drill.

5. Powered drills that are run continuously may heat the bone to 50°C, causing irreversible necrosis and reabsorption.

> **Key points**
>
> • When overheated bone dies and is reabsorbed; inserted screws loosen.
> • Drill intermittently for short periods.
> • Cool the bit with cold, sterile, physiological saline.

6. Once a hole is drilled it may be enlarged using a reamer (OE = to make room). Various shaping bits can be used, as when preparing a joint socket for replacement.
7. The availability of accurately made prostheses (G *pros* = to + *thesis* = a putting; hence an addition to or substitution of, for example, lost parts), demands that they are accurately fitted. When fixing bones by screwing on metal plates and similar devices, you must drill the holes accurately both for perfect alignment and also to avoid excessively weakening the bone. Whenever possible make use of drill guides (Fig. 8.13). For many standardized procedures special drill guides form part of the kit to enable you to drill screw holes accurately.
8. Clear away bone chips after drilling a hole.

> **Key points**
>
> • Control drills; protect the soft tissues; protect your eyes.
> • Repeatedly check that the exit is free from tissues that could be damaged or caught up.
> • Do not angle drills – the bits are brittle and will break.
> • Do not exert excessive pressure or you will jam the bit.

FIXING

Screws

1. Properly used, screws are very versatile and provide a valuable method of fixing bones, and for fixing plates and prostheses to bone.
2. Screws are made from a variety of metals including stainless steel, vitallium or titanium. Pure titanium provokes almost no tissue reaction and also does not interfere with magnetic resonance imaging (MRI). Biodegradable screws, usually of long chain polymers, are not yet in general use.
3. When using metals, ensure that they are compatible. If screws of one metal hold plates of another metal they generate electrolytic action, weakening the metal and provoking bone absorption.

> **Key points**
>
> • Do not screw cortical bone as you screw cancellous bone or wood, which accept the extra volume of a screw by compacting.
> • Cortical bone is already compact and is brittle. Provide an adequate hole or it will split.

4. Screws differ according to the function they are intended to perform (Fig. 8.14). Those that need a firm grip of the dense cortex have a thicker stem and short strong threads. Those that are inserted into the less dense cancellous bone have a slimmer stem and wider, thinner threads, since they can compact and grip the medullary inner bone. It is conventional to

Fig. 8.14 A Cortical screws are usually inserted through both the near and far cortex of, for example, a long bone. For this reason the hole is normally drilled and tapped so it grips at both ends. The screw end is rounded so that its projecting tip does not potentially damage soft tissue beyond. A cortical screw cannot be self-drilling because the sharp edge of the tip is blunted by the first cortex and cannot penetrate the second one. **B** Cortical screws may be self-tapping but the bevelled tapping tip must project far enough for the full succeeding thread to engage within the distal cortex. **C** Cancellous screws have narrower shafts but wider threads in order to compact and grip the looser cancellous bone. They are self-tapping and are not intended to enter and grip the distal cortex. **D** A self-drilling and self-tapping cancellous screw has a fluted sharp-edged tip that cuts a thread as the screw is inserted. This facilitates percutaneous insertion, increasingly valuable with modern techniques. **E** Cancellous screws may have a thread formed only at the distal end of a screw while the proximal shaft remains smooth. This is a lag screw. If it crosses a gap before re-entering cancellous bone and is then tightened it closes the gap. **F** When it is difficult to align a screw correctly, insert a guidewire, check that it is correctly positioned and pass a cannulated screw over it and screw it in before withdrawing the guidewire. **G** A screw fixing a plate to bone may then be solidly fixed to the plate. The screw head is threaded and engages with an internal thread on the inside of the hole. The screw is cancellous, self-tapping. It does not penetrate the far cortex because the cutting edge is lost on the near cortex.

5. Lag screws have smooth shafts near the head and screw threads only on the distal portion. The intention is that the thread draws whatever it enters tightly up against the material near the proximal part (see later).

6. It may be difficult to place a screw correctly and one method of avoiding an error is to insert guidewires until one proves to be correct. A cannulated screw can be fed over the guidewire and screwed in, after which the guidewire is withdrawn. Screws holding bone plates can be locked to the plate by having a threaded screw head which engages with an internal thread in the plate hole (see later).

7. If a cortical screw is inserted across a longitudinally split long bone and tightened, it will not close the gap (Fig. 8.15). If the proximal cortex is drilled oversize so that the threads in the proximal cortex do not engage, the threads in the distal cortex draw the separated bones together. Do not attempt to employ a cancellous screw with a smooth proximal shaft for this because the distal cancellous screw threads will not grip the dense distal cortex.

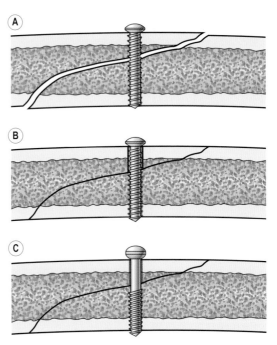

Fig. 8.15 A A fully threaded screw inserted in a fully tapped track created while the bones remain apart will have no compression effect on the gap. **B** If the proximal cortex is drilled oversize, the screw acts as a lag screw, compressing the bones. **C** Do not use a cancellous screw, with an unthreaded part of the shank, as an alternative to drilling the proximal fragment oversized and using a cortical screw. The cancellous screw will not grip the far cortex sufficiently securely.

drill a hole, tap the hole and finally insert the screw for cortical screws but cancellous screws are able to cut their own threads through the softer bone. Self-tapping cortical screws have increased in popularity since many are now inserted percutaneously. Self-drilling and self-tapping screws exist but these must not be used if the screw is intended to grip the far cortex, since the cutting edges are destroyed as they pass through the near cortex.

8. When fixing long bones, the specialized screws must pierce and grip the dense outer bone, usually of both cortices; these are cortical screws and are threaded along their whole length. First drill a hole of the same bore as the shank of the screw from which the thread flanges project. Measure the length of the hole so you can select the correct length of screw. Now use a tap of the correct size to cut the thread. Unscrew the tap, remove the loose bony fragments and insert the screw (Fig. 8.16).

> ### Key points
>
> - Do not over-tighten screws; if you do, you will strip the threads.
> - Perform the final tightening with finger and thumb pressure on the screwdriver.

9. If you place a screw perpendicular to the bone surface to unite oblique surfaces in a long bone, such as a fracture line, it will slip when longitudinal stresses are applied. Instead, insert the screw perpendicular to the fracture line (Fig. 8.17). In practice the single screw will not stabilize the fracture, so it will usually be supported by a plate and screws; these plate-holding screws are inserted at right angles to the bone and do not cross the fracture (see later).

10. If there is a spiral fracture, insert the screws through the middle of the fragments along the bone, so they also form a spiral (Fig. 8.18).

11. If a screw-head protrudes and will interfere with function, cause pain or be unsightly, use a countersink drill bit to create a depression into which the screw head fits.

12. Sometimes retained screws and other metal inserts, such as plates, cause problems after they have served their purpose and may need to be removed. The short- and long-term results of both glass ceramic and biodegradable screws are under trial.

Stitching

Stitches can be inserted into periosteum or ligaments. Alternatively, you may drill holes into which you can insert stitches. Special small screws can be inserted into bone, which carry a thread. The thread can be used to attach a structure to the bone.

Fig. 8.16 Inserting a cortical screw. From above downwards: drill a hole through both cortices. Use a depth gauge to measure the required length of screw; tap the hole to cut the screw thread; insert and drive home the screw.

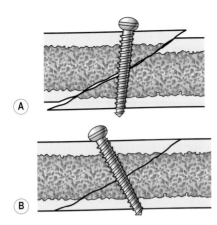

Fig. 8.17 **A** A screw inserted perpendicularly across the bone will not hold an oblique fracture, which will slip. **B** The screw must be perpendicular to the fracture and oblique to the shaft. Of course, a single screw would not suffice. If the fracture needs plating, the plate screws are inserted perpendicular to the bone.

Fig. 8.19 Wiring bone. **A** The ends of the encircling wire are evenly twisted. **B** One wire has been wound round the other wire, which is straight. This is insecure. **C** Drill the bone and pass wire through the holes in the manner of a stitch.

Fig. 8.18 Insert screws through the middle of the fragments to stabilize a spiral fracture, so they also form a spiral.

Wiring

1. Bone can be fixed by encircling it with wire (Fig. 8.19). This may prejudice the blood supply, so it is infrequently used for normal circumstances and the wire is often removed later.
2. Twist the wire ends evenly. If you keep one end straight and wrap the other around it, it has no holding power. If you over-tighten the wire it will fracture. Turn the ends of the twisted wire so they do not protrude under the skin or press upon vulnerable structures.
3. As an alternative to encircling wire, drill holes through the bone and use wire like a stitch.
4. In some situations the bone can be stapled, especially if it is cancellous. Tap in the staple in an introducer, then remove the introducer so the staple can be driven fully home.
5. Encircling wire fixation is finding an increasing use as patients with longstanding prosthetic joints develop peri-prosthetic fractures. Screw fixation of plates may not be possible but special screws with eyed heads can be screwed into plate holes so that encircling wires can be attached to the eyes and tightened to fix the plate.

Plates

1. Metal plates are manufactured of stainless steel, vitallium and titanium (Fig. 8.20). They may be straight, angled flat, tubular, with round or oval holes, holes arranged in rows or staggered. It is now recognized that the pressure of the plate tends to crush the delicate periosteum and occlude the blood supply to the underlying bone. Whenever possible, use low contact plates which are undercut between the screw holes.
2. Plates may be used as struts to maintain mechanical support or as buttresses pushing in a fragment (Fig. 8.21).
3. At operation place the bones in correct alignment, select a suitable-sized plate and if necessary bend it to fit accurately. Make sure that at least three holes lie over each fragment.

Fig. 8.20 **A** Various metal plates. **B** Side view of low contact plate designed to reduce pressure on the periosteum.

Fig. 8.21 Plate used as a buttress to hold a fragment in place.

4. Clamp the plate in place while drilling though the centre of each hole towards the opposite cortex, using a drill guide.

Key points

- Do not overstrip the peritoneum or crush it. When possible, use low-contact plates.
- Be very careful not to splinter the bone as the drill emerges at the opposite cortex and so prejudice the grip of the screw on the cortex.
- Protect soft tissues from damage by the emerging drill bit.

5. Estimate the required screw lengths using a depth gauge. Tap the holes and insert the screws (Fig. 8.22). Do not over-tighten them.

Fig. 8.22 Plating and screwing long bone. Ensure that the plate lies in contact along its length. From top to bottom, drill a hole through both cortices; measure the required screw length using a depth gauge; tap the hole; insert the screw, which should grip the opposite cortex as well as the near one.

6. You may not have access to the ends of the bone on the opposite side from the fracture. If they are not in contact, the plate bridging the break becomes a fulcrum when bone comes under tension; the bone ends are alternatively compressed and retracted on the side opposite the plate, causing reabsorption and preventing union. Make sure to check for a gap with X-rays.

7. *Compressing* the separated ends of the bone facilitates union. A simple method of achieving this is to use compression plates with longitudinally oriented oval holes. As the round-headed screw is tightened into the hole it distracts the plate, effectively shortening it (Fig. 8.23). If the other end of the plate has been firmly fixed to the other fragment, the result is to draw the bones together.

8. A special compression plate can be used. First securely anchor one end on one side of the break. Apply the other component, crossing over the break (Fig. 8.24), so that the hook on the fully opened anchored section can engage in the nearest screw hole. Fix the second plate at its far end from the compression device. Now tighten the screw to draw the two parts together. Insert intermediate screws on both sides of the break. Finally, release the compression device, unscrew it and insert the final screw in the plate that had been engaged with the compression device hook.

Fig. 8.23 As the round-headed screw-head is tightened into the oval hole in the plate, it produces distraction.

Fig. 8.24 Compression plate. Firmly fix the compression device on the right. Place the plate, crossing the break, so the hook on the fully opened compression device fits into the last screw hole. Fix the opposite end of the plate. Tighten the compression device. Place intermediate screws on both sides of the break. Slacken off and remove the compression device before inserting the last screw in the hole formerly occupied by the hook of the compression device.

Fig. 8.26 An external fixator.

Fig. 8.25 Mechanism of locked plate. As the screws are driven through the plate and into bone, the screw thread on the head of the screws engages with the threaded hole in the plate, locking it and fixing the bone and plate. Note that the plate does not need to be in contact with bone everywhere along its length.

9. *Locked plate* fixation is a major advance offering some of the advantages of external fixation. The plate does not need to be in close contact with bone throughout the whole length and can bridge partial gaps, reducing the need for muscular and periosteal stripping. Unicortical screws suffice since they have threads on their heads which engage with screw threads cut into the plate holes; when fully engaged, they grip the bone and are also locked to the plate (Fig. 8.25). The procedure can be partly accomplished by sliding the plate down through an incision under imaging control. Some of the locking screws can be inserted percutaneously through small incisions. The effect is similar to that of external fixators, with pins locking the bones on each side of the break and holding them in a firm relationship with each other.

External fixators

1. Many of these are complex and require advanced skills in order to employ them. Consequently they are described only to outline the principles on which they work. An important advantage is that the site of

a break in continuity can be left undisturbed, fixation being undertaken at a distance on each side.

2. Two or more threaded pins are inserted percutaneously, through small local incisions, into the bone on either side of the break, and at a distance from it. The pins can then be fixed with clamps at each site. After ensuring, usually with radiological confirmation, that the fragments are perfectly aligned, the clamps are locked onto a common external linkage (Fig. 8.26). The fixators can be adjusted and then relocked if necessary, and the distance between the two groups of fixing pins can be reduced or increased to compress or distract the ends. A more stable arrangement is for the pins to pass right through the limb so the projecting ends can be attached to a second fixator.

3. During the 1950s, G. A. Ilizarov in Kurgan, Siberia, developed a system of transfixing the bones above and below a break, using wires crossed at right angles to each other, attached under tension across external metal rings. The rings are linked across the break by rods and can be adjusted with turnbuckles to compress or distract the ends. The versatility of the method was further extended by the spatial frame developed by Taylor, allowing realignment by finely adjusting the turnbuckles on the six oblique struts to alter the relation of the rings (Fig. 8.27).

Intramedullary fixation

1. Smooth, double-pointed wires of various lengths and diameters were invented by Martin Kirschner, Professor of Surgery in Heidelberg, in 1909. They can be driven through bone with a T-handled chuck or a powered drill (Fig. 8.28) and inserted percutaneously or introduced at operation. Use a single wire to fix small bones such as phalanges by impaling them as though on a skewer. A number of fragments can be threaded on the wire like a kebab (Fig. 8.29). Use the largest size you can insert without splitting the fragments. Insert several wires in order to prevent rotation of the fragments (Fig. 8.30). Kirschner wires

Fig. 8.28 A powered drill to insert wires.

Fig. 8.29 Impaled fragments of a phalanx on a Kirschner wire.

Fig. 8.27 The Taylor Spatial Frame is a versatile development of the Ilizarov method of fixation of fractures. Tensed cross wires within the upper two rings form a stable base for the proximal bone and the lower single ring can be adjusted to align the distal bone correctly by changing the lengths of the adjustable struts.

offer a valuable method of stabilizing fragments while you apply permanent fixation.

2. An early intramedullary fracture fixation was the trifin nail for femoral neck fractures developed in 1931 by the Norwegian American Marius Smith-Peterson.

Femoral neck and intertrochanteric region are now usually treated using a large cancellous lag screw which engages with the cancellous bone of the femoral head. The smooth proximal shaft of the screw slides within a tube fixed to a plate screwed to the femoral shaft. As the screw is tightened it compresses the neck but as weight-bearing further compresses the fracture the screw can slide within the tube. It is thus dynamic (G *dynasthai* = to be able) as opposed to static (Fig. 8.31), producing a stabilizing compression effect.

Fig. 8.30 Insert Kirschner wires to prevent rotation of the fragments.

(A) (B) (C) (D)

Fig. 8.31 The principle of the lag screw to compress and stabilize a fractured neck of femur. **A** A guidewire is passed and the correct depth is calculated. **B** The track is drilled out. **C** The section external to the break is reamed out, while the section internal to the break is tapped. **D** A lag screw type of pin is screwed into the inner fragment, and a plate is fixed to the shaft of the femur, carrying a tube within which the shaft of the lag screw can slide and rotate, producing a dynamic hip screw.

3. The intramedullary nail for femoral shaft fractures was developed by Gerhard Küntscher of Kiel in 1940. In many long bones intramedullary nails can be inserted, often through the metaphysis and with minimal exposure, then locked with screws or pins introduced percutaneously through the bone and holes at each end of the nail, to prevent rotation. Especially for children, flexible titanium nails can be inserted, usually avoiding damage to the metaphysis (Fig. 8.32).

Bone grafts

1. Cancellous (L *cancelli* = lattice-work, hence, spongy, porous) bone has little strength but has osteogenic potential. A convenient site is the iliac crest. Expose it, detach the external muscles and cut across the crest with an osteotome, leaving it still attached to the internal muscles. Cut thin slices from the exposed edge. Remove the exposed cancellous bone using a gouge, leaving the inner cortex intact. Finally replace the iliac crest and secure it by suturing the muscles over it (Fig. 8.33).
2. Cortical bone is strong and can be fixed in place. It is, though, slowly vascularized, may be reabsorbed and has little osteogenic potential. It can be used as a support or strut, to fill a gap.
3. Autografts (G *autos* = self) are usually used. Allografts (G *allos* = other; from other humans, usually by donation) that are free from viral infection can be used intact or morselized (chopped), obtained from bone banks, or stimulated by bone morphogenetic proteins.

AMPUTATION

1. Plan amputation (L *ambi* = around + *putare* + to prune) distal to a joint in order to preserve joint function if possible. Aim to retain the muscle insertions into the distal stump. Preserve sufficient length of stump if you wish to fit a prosthesis onto it.
2. As a rule fashion flaps of healthy skin with underlying tissue, retracted to expose the bone. Single or double flaps are used depending on the vitality and vascularity of the tissues. Divide the fully exposed bone with a saw after protecting all the soft tissues. Establish perfect haemostasis. Smooth the bone stump using a rasp.
3. Close the flaps over the stump (Fig. 8.34). Monitor the stump vitality carefully until it is fully healed.
4. Amputation can often be avoided when a length of long bone must be removed for some tumours. After excising the diseased bone, the defect can sometimes be bridged with a graft or metal prosthesis, leaving the limb intact.
5. A method of attaching a prosthesis to an amputated limb has been developed after studying the annual growth and shedding of antlers in deer. A metal terminal prosthesis implanted into the distal end of the transected bone carries a screw end that protrudes through the skin. A porous ring lying just beneath the skin allows a natural seal to form, preventing bacterial invasion. A prosthesis can be attached to the protruding screw.

Fig. 8.32 A A rigid intramedullary nail; at each end screws or pins can be driven through holes in the nail to prevent rotation. **B** Two flexible titanium nails have been introduced. The curvatures impinge on the inner cortex in the middle of the shafts and hold the fractured ends in contact.

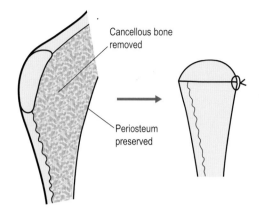

Cancellous bone removed

Periosteum preserved

Fig. 8.33 Harvesting cancellous bone. Elevate the iliac crest like the lid of a box, remove cancellous bone, then replace and suture the crest.

Fig. 8.34 Amputation. This shows a below-knee amputation. Leave the tibia sufficiently long so that a prosthesis can be fitted to it and the knee can be controlled by the descending muscles. The posterior flap has been kept long so that it can be brought over the bone end and stitched to the short anterior flap. Note the rounding of the anterior edge of the tibia.

Joints

1. Many operations are now carried out on joints using arthroscopy. An intra-articular space is created by distending the joint with normal saline. Different parts of the joint may be made accessible by moving the joint during examination or operative procedure.
2. The hyaline cartilage covering bone ends engaging in synovial joints is avascular and nourished by diffusion, so it has a limited ability to repair itself if it is diseased or damaged. Intra-articular tears of the meniscal cartilage in, for example, the knee, can be smoothed or repaired, especially near the periphery, which is adjacent to the blood supply. Partial meniscectomy may be necessary but if possible total meniscectomy is avoided because of the risk of eventual arthritis. Developments are underway for replacing the meniscus.
3. The capsule surrounding synovial joints is composed of tough fibrous tissue and this is in places thickened into ligaments which stabilize the joint and limit its movements. Unlike tendons, ligaments are elastic and

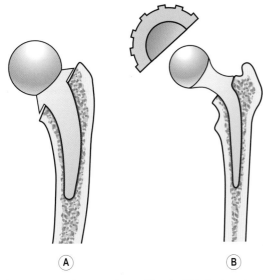

Fig. 8.35 A Replacement femoral head which fits into the acetabulum. **B** Total hip replacement. The replacement head fits into a socket fixed into the reamed out acetabulum.

will stretch if subjected to continuous tension exerted accidentally as following an uncorrected dislocation, or deliberately, to increase joint mobility.

4. A torn intra-articular ligament such as the anterior cruciate ligament of the knee may be removed and replaced. Prosthetic synthetic materials may be used or allografts (G *allos* = other – from another species). Autografts (G *autos* = self) are commonly used of two types (see later).
5. Certain joints or joint elements can be replaced when they are diseased or damaged.
6. For some fractures of the hip the best treatment may be replacement of the femoral head and neck with a metal prosthesis. The new head and neck are fixed into the femoral medullary cavity by means of a metal stem (Fig. 8.35). Stem fixation may be achieved using polymethylmethacrylate cement or the stem surface can be coated, for example with sintered metal beads to encourage direct bonding with the tissues, which grow around the beads, providing a solid fix.
7. For complete hip replacement, the acetabulum (L = vinegar cup) is reamed out to enlarge it and a cup is inserted to receive the replacement femoral head. The head may be of metal, plastic material or ceramic; this has a low wear rate and its former brittleness has now been overcome. Ultra high molecular weight polyethylene (UHMWPE) articulating with metal may be a successful combination.
8. Other joints can be successfully replaced, or the contacting surfaces can be replaced. Small joints, such as those in the fingers, can be replaced using one-piece flexible, usually Silastic, prostheses.

CARTILAGE

1. The articulating ends of bones are covered with hyaline cartilage. If it is damaged it may sometimes be repaired; if it heals, this is with fibrocartilage. Healing is more certain the nearer the damage lies in relation to the blood supply, since cartilage is avascular and intra-articular. In some joints, notably the knee, there are cartilagenous menisci between the bone ends. The contacting surfaces can be smoothed. This is usually achieved arthroscopically.
2. Various techniques are used in the hope of replacing deficient articular cartilage, such as creating multiple perforations in the bone, with the hope that the underlying bone marrow contains pluripotent cells that can reproduce the cartilage; alternatively, periosteum contains pluripotent cells. Multiple cartilage-covered bone grafts may be laid down.

LIGAMENTS

1. These unite bone to bone, preventing or restricting movement. In many joints they may form part of the surrounding capsule.
2. When subjected to increased tension over a period, ligaments stretch, especially in youth, permitting an increased range of movement.
3. Ligaments around the knee are particularly at risk of damage. Lateral trauma tends to open the knee joint medially and so tear the medial collateral ligament.
4. A twisting motion, especially when the foot is firmly on the ground, may rupture the anterior cruciate ligament. Women are more at risk than are men. Operative repair is not always necessary. In some cases the tear can be sutured. Removal and replacement may be carried out. In one method, braided hamstring tendons are led between the tibia and the femur. Alternatively, the central section of the patellar ligament, with attached bone from the patella and the tibia, may be used, since the bone fragments at each end will fuse with the femur above and the tibia below.

TENDON INSERTION

1. If a tendon ruptures at its insertion into bone it is usual practice to cut out a cortical panel so that it can be inserted into cancellous bone and sutured in after drilling stitch holes through which can be passed non-absorbable stitches.
2. If a distal stump of well-vascularized tendon remains, unite the ends.

Chapter | 9 |

Handling dissection

Dissection (L *dis* = apart + *secare* = to cut) may be necessary to approach a structure to identify, display, examine, repair or resect it. It demands an intimate knowledge of the anatomy and the differential make-up of tissues in health and disease. One of the hallmarks of surgical competence is the ability to carry out dissection in the presence of unusual conditions. For this reason patients with complications from previous operations, those with difficult and extensive diseases and those with co-morbidity tend to be referred to surgeons who are recognized to have exceptional competence. They did not acquire the competence by chance but by outstanding concentration and effort.

ORGANIZE

1. Ensure that the patient is in the position that facilitates exposure – supine, prone, straight or flexed.
2. If necessary have the operating table tilted, provided the patient is properly secured.
3. Make use of gravity; for example, when operating in the pelvis, to empty it of bowel, place the patient head down (the position named after the German surgeon Friedrich Trendelenburg, 1844–1925). Alternatively, place the patient head up to ensure that the neck veins are not congested when operating on the neck (often

called 'reversed Trendelenburg'). Raise limbs to reduce congestion.

4. Place pillows or sandbags to elevate a part or retain the patient in the required posture.
5. In some cases ensure that you can turn the patient or limb during the procedure.
6. Ensure that you have good, shadowless, glare-free light. When appropriate, make use of light-carrying retractors and headlight.

EXPOSE

1. Plan the incision carefully. Do not compromise on attaining safe access but consider the cosmetic and functional effects. Many generations of surgeons have accumulated a wealth of standardized safe approaches. Use a standard approach whenever possible but remember that there are anatomical anomalies and also that disease processes may change the anatomy. In addition, many standard approaches have caveats (L *cavere* = to take care), such as the need to avoid entering the brachial artery when giving an intravenous injection at the elbow, and to avoid injury to the facial nerve when operating on the parotid gland. If you need to use a novel method, study the anatomy carefully, asking yourself why your approach is not normally used.
2. In some cases you cannot predict the findings and may need to extend the incision, so adjust your incision to accommodate this. For limb surgery, A. K. Henry, Professor of Anatomy in Cairo, used the term 'extensile exposure' in his book on limb surgery,[1] meaning approaches that can be enlarged.
3. Make sure you are in the correct tissue layer – failure to do so may lead you into error.
4. When possible gently split muscle and aponeurotic fibres rather than cut them. You may be able to displace nerves, blood vessels, tendons and ligaments rather than transect them.
5. Make use of the full length of the incision and if necessary, have the wound edges retracted. Prefer dynamic retraction by an assistant, which can be adjusted as necessary and relaxed at intervals, to fixed self-retaining retraction. Your assistant can gently displace intervening structures with fingers, after covering slippery tissues with a gauze swab (Fig. 9.1). Apply tissue forceps to tough structures to retract them (Fig. 9.2).
6. Make use of gravity by moving the patient or a part to displace an obstructing, intervening structure. Alternatively use large packs with tapes attached to substantial metal rings kept outside the wound or clipped to the external towels, to guard against leaving them inside (Fig. 9.3). Sometimes a structure cannot be removed but can be rotated on its anchoring tissues; for example, the left lobe of the liver can be

Fig. 9.1 Retracting with fingers over a gauze swab to improve the grip on slippery tissues.

Fig. 9.2 Use tissue forceps to retract tough tissues.

gently folded to give access to the oesophageal hiatus, and the column of trachea, larynx, oesophagus and thyroid gland can be rotated to bring the posterior aspect of the pharynx into view.

7. Prefer to bring a mobile structure to the surface of the wound in preference to carrying out a delicate procedure in the depths where the lighting and access are limited. Sometimes a pack can be placed beneath a structure to raise it (Fig. 9.3); alternatively try depressing the edges of the incision (Fig. 9.4).

Key points

- Exposure is prejudiced by poor haemostasis. Blood staining obscures the distinctive appearance of differing tissues.
- If you wish to see what you are doing, first stop the bleeding.

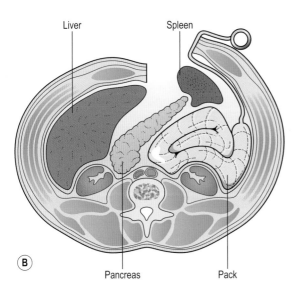

Fig. 9.3 Large packs. **A** The pack holds aside a structure to prevent it from intruding into the wound, in this case small bowel loops. **B** A large pack placed behind a structure lifts it up into the mouth of the wound. Note the tapes attached to large metal rings left outside the wound.

Fig. 9.4 Displaying a fixed deep structure. As an alternative to retracting the wound edges, as in **A**, is it possible to depress them as in **B**?

Fig. 9.5 If you apply tension to separate the margins of the incision when cutting with a scalpel, you display the depths of the wound, so you do not inadvertently cut too deeply.

DISSECTION METHODS

Sharp

1. The scalpel divides tissues with the minimum damage. If the tissues move under the drag of the scalpel steady them with your fingers, if necessary separating your fingers to open up the incision, displaying the deeper structures (Fig. 9.5).

2. Expertly performed scissors dissection produces minimal damage especially when floppy tissue is difficult to stabilize for cutting with a scalpel. Do not use blunt or loosely hinged scissors. The blades

151

Fig. 9.6 When cutting with scissors, protect the underlying structures from inadvertent damage by the deep blade.

must remain in contact or they tend to chew through the tissues. Scissors have the advantage that they can be used for blunt or sharp dissection. Insert the closed blades and gently open them to define a plane of cleavage, or cut the tissues to separate them. A potential danger is that the deep blade is hidden in some circumstances (Fig. 9.6), so first carefully inspect and palpate the deep surface.

Blunt

1. Splitting is a valuable method of dissecting in muscle, aponeuroses, and to open up tissues along the direction of linear structures such as vessels, nerves and tendons. It is a method that allows you to follow a natural path rather than creating one by sharp dissection. The line of cleavage is parallel to the strong fibres, which are held together by weaker interconnecting fibres. Scissors can be used to split a sheet after it has been penetrated in one place and separated from deep structures. Insert one blade of almost fully closed scissors into the hole and push them in the direction of the fibres (Fig. 9.7).
2. A different splitting action can be achieved with scissors by holding them perpendicular to the plane of the tissues. Push the closed tips between the fibres and gently open the blades (Fig. 9.8). Alternatively use artery forceps instead of scissors, since the tips have gently rounded backs. Even more gentle splitting can be achieved by inserting closed dissecting forceps and allowing them to open; the force is limited by the

Fig. 9.7 Splitting parallel fibres with scissors. Almost close the scissors and push the small 'V' between the blade tips into the tissues, along the line of the fibres.

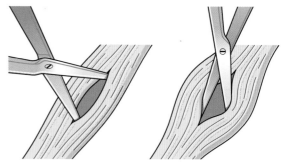

Fig. 9.8 Splitting parallel fibres with scissors. Push the closed tips into the sheet of tissue and open them parallel to the fibres. If there are underlying structures with side branches, open the scissors at right angles to the line of the intended split.

spring of the blades. The handle of a scalpel makes a convenient splitting instrument in some situations.

3. Tearing may seem to be a traumatic method, and so it can be if employed inappropriately or roughly. Used judiciously it allows you to find the line of weakness, perhaps when two structures are adherent and you do not wish to risk sharp dissection in case you inadvertently cut into one of them. Try inserting two fingers and gently separate them (Fig. 9.9); you have a very accurate feel of the force you are exerting. As you pull the tissues apart, feel and watch carefully to ensure the path of the separation does not deviate.

> **Key point**
>
> • Always apply distraction force as closely as possible to the line of separation.

4. Peeling is valuable when a flexible structure must be detached from another along an adherent tissue plane. Depending on the shape of the attachment, you may use a gauze pledget held in forceps (Fig. 9.10), a fingertip (Fig. 9.11), a fingertip wrapped with a gauze swab (Fig. 9.12) or a swab held in the fingers (Fig. 9.13). Peeling is not wiping, which traumatizes the tissues. If you need to wipe your way through the tissues, you do not know your anatomy. Occasionally you need to use a wiping action to grip by friction something you wish to wipe away from a surface provided this does not abrade the surface.
5. Pinching is sometimes valuable when you cannot obtain a view of an attachment in the depths of the wound. You may not be able to view the line of cleavage but by gently pinching the union you can assess the line of fusion (Fig. 9.14) and may be able to pinch it off (Fig. 9.15). The manoeuvre enables you, for example, to detach a benign gastric ulcer that is adherent to, or penetrating, another structure.

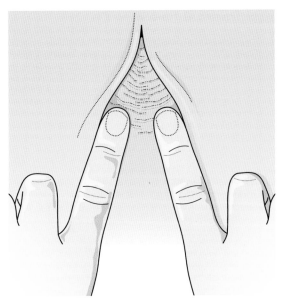

Fig. 9.9 Judicious separation of tissue by a tearing action, trying to sense the correct line of separation.

Fig. 9.11 Peeling off a structure using the tip of a finger.

Fig. 9.10 Using a pledget of gauze held in forceps to peel an adhesion.

Fig. 9.12 Wrap a finger with gauze to peel structures.

6. Finger fracture of solid organs sounds crude but when expertly performed it is an effective and safe method of splitting a bulky organ such as the liver. The split must be through healthy tissue because the consequences of compressing diseased tissues is unknown and could be disastrous. The scaffold matrix of connective tissues, vessels and ducts remain intact while the parenchymal cells are dislodged and disrupted (G *para* = beside + *enchyma* = an inpouring – from an ancient belief that the essential tissue cells were poured in and congealed). The vessels and ducts remain intact, crossing the created gap, and

153

Fig. 9.13 To give you a frictional grip in peeling off a larger structure, hold a gauze swab in your hand.

Fig. 9.14 Gently pinch the junction to assess it if you cannot easily visualize it.

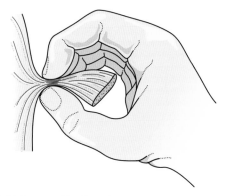

Fig. 9.15 By a combined pinching and peeling action from both sides simultaneously, you may be able to separate the tissues safely.

can be identified, isolated, sealed electrosurgically or ultrasonically, clipped, sutured or double ligated with division between the ties. Because no heat has been applied with the finger compression, their structure is not weakened.

Instrumental (see also Ch. 2)

1. A long-established electrosurgical method of dissection is cutting diathermy, usually applied through a unipolar needle. A mixed cutting and coagulation current may be used to seal blood vessels as they are cut. Bipolar diathermy forceps allow small bites to be taken and sealed.

2. A Kelly haemostatic clamp used in gynaecology can be placed along the line of dissection, crushing and disrupting parenchymal cells but preserving vessels and ducts so they can be clipped and ligated or sealed with diathermy, in a similar method to finger fracture.

3. Ultrasound dissection usually at 20–30 kHz acts mainly by cellular cavitation and disruption of parenchymal cells. It can be applied by a rod or hook, leaving the vessels and ducts intact. The CUSA™ system incorporates an irrigation and suction facility to wash out and remove the dislodged debris. It is a valuable method of dissection in fragile tissue, as in ocular cataract phaco-emulsification and also in the brain. At higher frequencies such as 55.5 kHz, small bites of tissue can be compressed within a clamp, such as the Harmonic Scalpel®, so that vessels within it are flattened, coapting and coagulating the intima to seal them, before dividing them.

4. Tissue can be grasped, cauterized and then divided using the LigaSure™ electrosurgical system. It is activated on the tissue enclosed and compressed in the jaws, to melt the collagen and elastin to form a seal, then automatically switched off, when the tissues can be transected. It is claimed to seal vessels up to 7 mm diameter.

5. A high-pressure water jet also dislodges parenchymal cells while preserving other structures.

6. Lasers of different types are used to incise or destroy a variety of tissues but this requires special training, and careful regulation of the depth of penetration.

7. Cryosurgery is accomplished using liquid nitrogen to create an ice ball which eventually separates.

8. An argon plasma (ionized) beam created between an electrosurgical generator and the tissue surface allows the high-frequency electric current to flow, to coagulate and seal small vessels.

9. Radiofrequency thermal ablation can be carried out by implanting an electrode which produces ionic agitation and heating with destruction, before dissection.

LAYERED OR SOLID TISSUES?

The difference between dissecting within layers of tissue and sectioning a solid structure, such as a large organ, a large mass or an agglomeration of tissue forming a mass, is often unrecognized.

1. Layers can be separated into planes and each one then dealt with sequentially. By keeping in the correct plane at all times, the risk of inadvertent damage is minimized. You have access to the undersurface of each layer as well as the presenting surface.
2. When you enter a solid mass you have only the presenting surface available to examine directly. You must, from your anatomical, pathological, imaging and experiential knowledge, make a judgement of the underlying tissues within the mass.
3. Appreciate the difference between dissecting in layered and in solid tissues. Layered tissues can be separated and identified by feel, often by folding, to examine the deep surface. A light can be placed beneath successive layers to transilluminate them, so that vessels can be identified and ligated or sealed before dividing them. Solid tissue of indeterminate nature may be impossible to deal with by creating artificial layers, and must be divided from the surface while attempting to anticipate vital structures ahead.

Key points

- Anticipate, identify and react to the type of dissection required.
- Dissecting in diseased solid structures demands a surgeon with exceptional skill and experience.

The need for constant awareness of danger and supreme operative skill applies especially to dissections within structures like the brain and liver. It is particularly demanding during the extracapsular removal of a potentially invasive tumour, keeping outside the apparent plane of cleavage.

TISSUE PLANES

Key points

- This is, perhaps, the most neglected aspect of dissecting. Intimate knowledge of the correct plane distinguishes the master from the pedestrian surgeon.
- When the anatomy is distorted, once you confidently reach the surface of an identified structure, do not lightly wander from it, because you are then entering an unknown area.

1. For example, when operating on the thyroid gland you need to pick up sequential diaphanous layers of fascia with two pairs of fine forceps and incise between them, until you see the veins on the gland fill up as the last restraint is removed, confirming that you have entered the correct plane. Similarly when exposing the abdominal oesophagus at the hiatus

you need to incise the peritoneum and then the phreno-oesophageal ligament. Dissecting in the limbs requires you to know and follow the structures in relation to each other so you can reach your target site with minimal damage to others; A. K. Henry, who was Professor of Anatomy in Cairo, beautifully described classic limb exposures.[1]
2. When you are dissecting near the liver, for example, do not lightly wander from it. It is a valuable marker; its surface is a tissue plane you can follow to reach contiguous structures safely.
3. When opening up an obliterated tissue plane you may know the structure and the strength of the structure on one surface, but do not assume the strength of the tissues that you are separating from it, so take great care until you have confirmed its nature.
4. When dissecting along a structure such as a nerve or blood vessel, proceed carefully to avoid damaging any branches, tributaries or other structures. Nerves, arteries, veins and lymphatics often run in parallel.
5. The greatest challenge is to leave the safe plane in order to encompass tissues, such as an infiltrating malignant tumour, that must be excised together with a surrounding layer of healthy tissue. The difficulty is two-fold: you must know the normal anatomy and the possible results of distortion, and you must be able to distinguish normal tissue from potentially malignant tissue.

Key points

- If disease has distorted the anatomy, do not inexorably persist in your intended approach. Try approaching it from different aspects.
- Also, try starting your dissection from a short distance away in normal tissue and work towards the diseased area.

6. Membranous layers often overlie important structures and you may find it impossible to be sure if the underlying structures are attached until you have breached the layer. If the membrane is sufficiently lax, pinch up a fold with your fingers to estimate its thickness and mobility on underlying structures by rolling it between your fingers. Now pick up a fold with dissecting forceps to tent it. Apply a second forceps close by on the tented portion, release and reapply the first forceps to allow anything caught in its initial grasp of untented membrane to fall away. Have the two forceps held up to create a raised ridge. Make a small scalpel incision on the crest of the ridge to let air enter and allow any structure to fall away (Fig. 9.16). This is a standard technique when opening the peritoneum in abdominal operations.

155

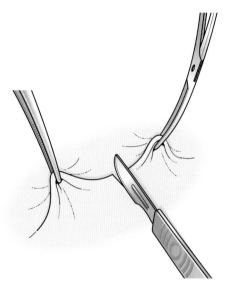

Fig. 9.16 Make an initial incision through a membrane after lifting a ridge with forceps.

7. Enlarge the incision so you can insinuate your finger and explore the undersurface of the membrane to ensure it is clear. Through the entry hole insert the blades of dissecting forceps, or two separated fingers, under the membrane and cut between them (Fig. 9.17). As you proceed it becomes progressively easier to inspect the deep aspect of the membrane.
8. When it is critically important to avoid cutting more than the membrane, infiltrate the layer with sterile physiological saline to expand the tissues and render them more translucent.
9. If the membrane is the peritoneum and it has been opened previously, always start the new incision just beyond the end of the previous closure where you can tent it and also reduce the risk of cutting an adherent

structure. If it is too tense to be tented, infiltrate it with saline to thicken it and allow you to estimate the residual thickness.
10. To divide a sheet of vascular tissue first doubly clamp major vessels before incising the membrane. The less tissue that is included in the ligatures, the less likely are they to be dislodged (Fig. 9.18). If there are few major vessels you may double clamp, divide and ligate sections (Fig. 9.19). Do

Fig. 9.18 Dividing a sheet of vascular connective tissue. Isolate and doubly clamp the vessels before incising the sheet.

Fig. 9.17 To enlarge a hole through a membranous layer, insert dissecting forceps through the hole and incise the membrane between the blades of the forceps, as indicated in the dotted line.

Fig. 9.19 Dividing a vascular membrane between haemostatic clips. The forceps on the right will not grip the full width of the flattened ribbon. On the left the portion of membrane has been bunched with dissecting forceps before clamping it. Note that the left-hand forceps have the tips projecting beyond the clamped membrane, to facilitate the application of a ligature.

not attempt to gather too large clumps within the forceps. Artery forceps grip well only near the tips. In addition, if vessels lie within bunched up tissue within a ligature, they can retract from the constricting ligature and rebleed.

11. If the sheet is very vascular, consider infiltrating it with isotonic saline containing adrenaline (epinephrine) in a concentration of 1:400 000 to produce vasoconstriction and reduce oozing. Alternatively, use cutting and coagulating diathermy current, or ultrasonic dissection.

SOLID TISSUES

The difficulty of such dissection is variable depending on the degree of homogeneity and the disease process necessitating the intervention.

Imaging

Modern imaging methods that help delineate deep-seated tumours are invaluable. Preoperative ultrasound (US) may now be studied in three dimensions in some units; intraoperative imaging partially compensates for the lack of the sense of touch, especially in minimal access techniques. Computerized tomography (CT) can produce three-dimensional views. Magnetic resonance imaging (MRI) with gadolinium contrast provides accurate information about the increased vascular network that results from the development of blood vessels within actively growing neoplasms.

Dissecting

1. Within large masses of lipomatous connective tissue, avoid over-confidence. Vital structures at risk may not be evident and are often also infiltrated with fat which both disguises and weakens them. Blood vessels may be torn and subsequently bleed.

2. Dissection is often necessary within a mainly healthy solid organ to reach a diseased area and is facilitated if the anatomy is well understood and conforms to expectations. The approach to the objective is sometimes signalled by slight changes resulting from reaction to the disease, including an apparent capsular effect because of expansion and resulting pressure. The presence of such a lesion may additionally distort the otherwise normal placement of ducts and blood vessels.

3. A particular difficulty is identifying the margins of a lesion within a solid organ when it has the same appearance and consistency as the normal tissues. The margin between the normal and abnormal may be indistinct, or in some cases what appears to be a margin or a capsule is not the real margin of the lesion; it may be compressed normal tissue resulting from expansion of the lesion, or it may be a capsule but neoplastic microscopic disease has passed through it.

4. Knowledge of segmental anatomy of some organs such as the liver and the lungs provides a means of resecting less of the healthy functioning organ than in the past. In the case of the lung, a single segment may be dissected out from the hilar artery, vein and bronchus. In the case of the liver the hilar vessels can be controlled by gently occluding them with a non-crushing clamp for up to 60 minutes at a time, described by James Hogarth Pringle in 1908. By freeing and rotating the liver, the hepatic veins can also be secured. The method of dissection can be finger fracture, crushing clamp, ultrasonic dissection using the Cavitron Ultrasonic Surgical Aspirator (CUSA®), electrosurgical, high-pressure water jet or other methods. Haemostasis may be achieved using conventional methods, argon beam diathermy and a fibrin glue such as Tisseel™ before apposing the raw surfaces.

5. If a mass consists of adherent structures which you must separate, it is likely that both the structures and the adhesions vary in strength. The force required to separate adhesions may cause tearing of important tissues, often requiring critically important selection and flexible choice of methods. It is in such circumstances that extremely delicate, controlled separation is required. You must be instantly aware of exactly where you are applying distraction, and be ready to stop instantly if there is any incipient tissue rupture.

6. The difficulty and danger is greatly increased if you need to encompass a lesion without encroaching on diseased tissues, as when performing a radical resection of a possible or confirmed malignant tumour. The presence of the tumour may distort the anatomy. You are creating a tissue plane through normal tissue, without inadvertently encroaching on the diseased tissues.

7. In the brain it may be difficult to differentiate between functionally vital and 'silent' areas of the cortex and in such cases it is usual to perform the operation under local anaesthesia so that functional or sensory loss can be anticipated. As you attempt to free the tumour, you may distort and tear vital areas or tracts. The pia mater is usually first sealed with bipolar diathermy before using a combination of bipolar diathermy and gentle suction to dissect into the brain, often using magnification. The Cavitron Ultrasonic Surgical Aspirator (CUSA®) is frequently employed as a dissecting instrument. If a plane of cleavage can be identified between normal and

abnormal brain, a gentle water jet may extend it in the same plane.

Occasionally a tumour cannot be removed completely for fear of causing damage to a vital structure or to a major blood vessel, including the superior sagittal sinus. Following accurate stereotactic (three-dimensional location) imaging, the residual tumour may respond to accurately focused radiotherapy or gamma knife surgery in which beams of radiation, each insufficient alone, intersect at one point and destroy the residual tumour.

8. A severe challenge is to re-explore a patient following a previous procedure of which you have no record, but which has failed or developed complications, or when the disease has recurred following a previous operation.

9. The ultimate challenge is to reoperate on patients who may have had a series of previous operations, perhaps when it is not clear what was found, what was attempted, what may or may not have been achieved, and what the nature of the deterioration that necessitates re-exploration is.

> ### Key points
>
> - Surgeons who specialize in reoperations that have failed or been followed by complications are at the pinnacle of professional competence.
> - They appear to have a sixth sense in anticipating nearby important structures. It is not magic. It is supreme familiarity with the appearance and feel of normal and diseased tissues.
> - You will not yet be called upon to repeat their accomplishments but try to acquire their sensitivity to incipient tissue changes and their expertise in dealing with them.
> - It will stand you in good stead.

10. Be flexible in the use of instruments for dividing the tissues. If you use a scalpel, scissors, diathermy, ultrasonic or other dissector, in the depths, you must try to detect in advance what you will uncover with each attempt to deepen the dissection and choose the appropriate instrument. Remember that electrosurgical and ultrasonic dissectors may cause heating effects in the tissues beyond the division, although the manufacturers claim that this is localized.

11. If possible separate the sides following an incision, to open it out and allow you to estimate the depth and quality of the remaining tissue. Make each successive cut along the line of the preceding one in the deepest part of the wound. Tentative, scratch-like cuts create ragged, oozing tags. The fibres are sometimes aligned predominantly in one direction. Try to split, rather than transect the fibres. If you are likely to encounter an important structure, prefer to dissect parallel to it rather than across it.

12. In some cases you may be able to take the full thickness in successive thin layers so you can identify important structures within each layer. As each successive layer is confirmed to be free from important structures you can then safely divide it. Create the layers by inserting the closed blades of scissors, artery forceps or dissecting forceps, then open the blades, or allow them to open, to create a space.

13. When seeking a structure within homogeneous tissue, it is often convenient to use a combined technique of cutting and blunt dissection. Remember, if you insert the closed blades of scissors or artery forceps and open them, the force at the tips of the blades is very high. Proceed slowly, inserting your finger to feel what is ahead.

14. Some structures vary in texture in different parts, especially in granularity. The breast often feels more dense in the axillary tail, the pancreas may feel more granular and solid in different areas. As a result it becomes difficult to differentiate lumpiness from lump. Fat also varies in texture in different areas.

> ### Key points
>
> - Whatever method you use to dissect, make sure you do not damage healthy tissues that will remain at the limit of your separation.
> - Damaged tissues are likely to break down, bleed, prejudice healing or become infected.
> - The last connection you cut to free the base of a tumour is the most likely to bring disaster unless you are very cautious.

DISEASED TISSUES

1. Take note of the changes as you approach an area of acute inflammation. Watch out for increased vascularity, oedema, tissue tension and fragility. Palpate the tissues as you proceed because the heat is immediately evident, even through your glove, especially on the dorsal surface of the second phalanx of your fingers. If the blood vessels are congested there is increased fluid filtration, with high protein, so raising the extracellular colloid osmotic pressure

and causing appreciable turgidity. Deliberately sniff in case you can detect a distinctive smell.

2. As you approach chronically inflamed tissues you may detect increasing fibrosis. You may also anticipate increased vascularity but this is not always evident.

3. Remember that it is not only infection that increases local vascularity – the vascular growth factors released by fast-growing neoplasms also generate increased vascularity and remarkable vasodilatation occurs in acute non-infective inflammatory diseases.

4. In chronic disease the fibrous tissue laid down in response to many disease processes is often irregular and opaque, so there is no warning of impending disaster. The connective tissue that normally encloses many important structures may be destroyed by disease. You may suddenly expose the structure and inadvertently damage it.

5. Disease often alters the character of the tissues so that they are not easily recognized. The anatomical features may be distorted, sometimes as a result of contraction of the fibrous tissue that has been laid down, as it matures. This effect is multiplied if the disease is chronic or recurrent, when there is successive deposition and reabsorption of fibrous tissue. Fibrous attachments sometimes draw out diverticula from hollow organs and ducts, which are in danger during dissection.

6. Remember that the differential strengths of tissues may be changed by disease processes. Tearing, splitting or pinching require you to anticipate which structure will give way. Be very cautious and sensitive to incipient tearing in an unexpected area. Structures that are normally swept aside confidently may be adherent, thickened and resistant to blunt dissection so that you may prefer sharp dissection.

7. Whenever possible, start the dissection in normal tissue away from the worst of the disease and work towards the diseased area, maintaining exposure and identification of important structures throughout.

NEOPLASMS

Key points

- Do your 'homework' beforehand. Do not hope for the best. Read, and reread, standard texts – your predecessors have recorded best approaches, likely and less likely findings, dangers, advice on avoiding errors – and recovery from errors.
- The basis of good management of neoplasms is built on the two pillars of anatomy and pathology.

1. If the tumour is a type that is known to be benign, or if biopsy or cytology has demonstrated this, you do not need to carry out wide excision. If it is encapsulated you can dissect close to the capsule and avoid damaging the surrounding structures.

2. Resection of a malignant neoplasm often demands dissection outside the normal planes in order to excise the tumour totally, along with associated channels of likely spread, for example along lymph channels and tissue planes. Become acutely sensitive to detect warning signs of impending encroachment on the neoplasm or of inadvertently damaging an important structure that should have been preserved. This can be extremely difficult but anticipate increasing vascularity, turgidity, fragility, fixation, fibrosis or prominent lymph nodes.

3. Some malignant neoplasms appear to be limited and perhaps encapsulated but tumour cells penetrate and extend outside the apparent tumour margins so you need to carry out an extracapsular excision, dissecting through normal tissues. Be aware that the surrounding structures may be displaced and infiltrated by the growth. In some cases the extent of the growth may be indefinite either on preoperative imaging or at operation. Neurosurgeons may find it impossible to detect the junction with surrounding normal tissue that can be excised and vital brain tissue that must be preserved.

4. Bulky tumours may be reduced using electrosurgery, laser, ultrasound and radiofrequency. Gynaecologists may destroy large fibroids in this manner to diminish their size and neurosurgeons reduce the bulk of, for example, posterior fossa tumours. Neurosurgeons occasionally debulk a tumour from within rather than try to dissect around a large mass which may be overlying a major structure including a blood vessel.

5. Do not squeeze the specimen as you gradually free it – you may be squeezing malignant cells into the bloodstream. If you are removing for diagnosis, crushing it will distort the specimen. Steady it by controlling contiguous and adventitious tissues.

6. If you think you may have encroached on unsuspected malignant tissue immediately stop and call in expert help and advice. If you carry on, your gloves and instruments may carry, and implant, malignant cells elsewhere.

AIDS TO DISSECTION

Anatomy

Learn the anatomy of the part. You must know the normal appearance and situation of the structures and the appearance, texture and relative strengths. It is disappointing that many trainee surgeons do not take the opportunity to revise the anatomy before every operation, whether they are performing it or assisting at it.

159

Palpation

If an important structure is likely to be palpable, feel for it before starting. It is valuable to make a habit of feeling the abdomen before starting an operation, when the abdominal wall is relaxed.

During the operation feel for arterial pulsations – but remember that tension may obliterate the pulse.

Key points

- Take every opportunity to feel normal and abnormal structures.
- Until you know the range of what is normal, you cannot confidently identify the abnormal.

Haemostasis

Keep the operative field clear of blood, which obscures the view and stains every structure the same colour. Bleeding is inimical to safe, effective dissection. Prevent potential bleeding, control it when it occurs and remove any blood that collects as a result of bleeding. Do not attempt to work in the depths, in a pool of blood, with continuing uncontrolled bleeding. This is a recipe for disaster. When you are operating on limbs you may use elevation and a tourniquet to produce a bloodless field (see Ch. 10), and you may position the patient to raise the operative field and prevent congestion of the veins.

Find a safe starting point

In some circumstances you can identify an initial structure that remains your guide.

1. When excising a parotid tumour, first identify the facial nerve emerging from the styloid foramen by developing the space just anterior to the tragus of the external ear. You can then follow it as it divides, and preserve it, and its branches.
2. Some vessels and nerves have reliable relationships to fixed structures and you can follow them from here. A well-known relationship is that of the long saphenous vein, which can be found reliably 5 cm (1½) above the tip of the medial malleolus of the tibia.
3. In the abdomen find a structure such as the liver edge, which you can follow. In the right iliac fossa you can find the base of the appendix by identifying the right paracolic gutter, the caecum and the ileocaecal union.

Tension

1. The ability to put tissues under tension is a valuable aid as a preliminary to dissection. It can be exerted by drawing structures apart with tapes, your hands or fingers, dissecting forceps, retractors, packs or tissue forceps (Fig. 9.20).
2. Judicious use of tension aids the identification of attachments, and the safest line of separation (Fig. 9.21). By varying the angle of traction you can judge the whole extent of the attachment and test

Fig. 9.20 Some methods of exerting traction. **A** Tape. **B** Fingers or hand. **C** Dissecting forceps. **D** Retractor. **E** Packs. **F** Tissue forceps.

Fig. 9.21 Use gentle traction to test the strength and view the line of attachment.

the strength in different areas, since most force is exerted at the edge opposite to the direction of angled traction (Fig. 9.22). As soon as an edge begins to separate, change the angle, so that you are constantly working round the attachment, aiming that the last separation takes place at the centre of the union.

3. Be willing to combine techniques. If you apply tension on one structure it may present an edge that you can peel down (Fig. 9.23). A combination of traction and sharp dissection is very effective (Figs 9.24, 9.25); as you draw one tissue from another, the connections can be examined and selectively divided. Keep changing your line of approach if you encounter difficulty.

Key point

- If you are applying tension to separate two structures, apply it as close as possible to the intended point of cleavage; the further the distance of your fingers from this, the less your control (see Ch. 1, p. 5 and Fig. 1.4).

Fig. 9.24 Combined use of tension and sharp dissection with a scalpel is very effective when the attachment is strong.

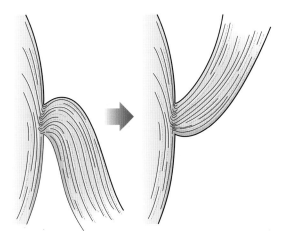

Fig. 9.22 Tension on the attachment is greatest at the point opposite the direction of traction, so you can observe the attachment round the whole circumference and plan the best site for attack.

Fig. 9.25 Gentle traction allows you to identify strong bands, which may be isolated and divided with scissors.

Dissecting around structures

1. You may need to dissect behind a large structure, either to secure the blood vessels entering and leaving it before excising it, or to carry out a procedure on another structure hidden behind the mass.
2. Ask yourself if you can avoid the problem by using another approach, or reduce the size of the mass – for example, deflate distended bowel or aspirate fluid from a cystic mass.
3. If you encounter difficulty, do not proceed doggedly on. Stop and reassess the problem. Can you approach

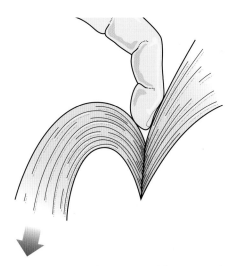

Fig. 9.23 Combined gentle traction and fingertip peeling will separate the two structures safely.

it from a different aspect, lengthen the incision, improve the retraction, improve the light, further mobilize the intervening structure?

4. Remember that the difficulty is usually greatest at the beginning. As you mobilize the target structure, exposure improves. However, do not forget that the other danger point is as you divide the final attachment, when you may become too casual and spoil a previously painstaking dissection.

5. Choose to start where you get the best view, where you are most confident about the anatomy, where you can best control blood vessels, and where a minor division of the tissues is likely to reap the highest rewards in facilitating further dissection. Of course, not all these aims are fulfilled at a single point, so choose the best compromise.

> **Key point**
>
> • Do not cut blindly. Failure to see is an indication for reassessment, not obsessive continuation.

6. Make sure that you have good control of potential bleeding. Remember, when trying to locate blood vessels, that applying tension is likely to obliterate arterial pulsations and empty veins so that you cannot identify them.

7. When transecting a pedicle underneath an overlying structure, it may be initially easier to transect it as far as possible from the mass but this may leave the remaining pedicle short and more difficult to secure (Fig. 9.26).

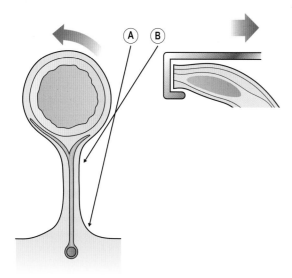

Fig. 9.26 The base of the pedicle is most easily seen at **A**, but the vessels can be better controlled if they are first sought at **B**.

Needles

If a sought-for structure is hard, as for example a stone, try locating it with the point of a sharp needle. Search for a cavity, duct or vessel containing fluid with a fine-bore hollow needle attached to a syringe to detect if you can aspirate identifiable fluid.

Fluid infiltration

In case of difficulty do not hesitate to infiltrate the tissues with isotonic saline to facilitate the separation of the structures. Fluid renders the tissues translucent, making it easier to see approaching structures. In some circumstances it is valuable to infiltrate the tissues with saline containing adrenaline (epinephrine) in a dilution of 1:200 000 in order to reduce oozing.

Transillumination

Sometimes the structures can be lifted and viewed against a light, or a light can be placed behind them. This allows you to view the vessels – but remember that compressed and emptied veins transilluminate. Always relax the tissues during transillumination. This method is very valuable when you are resecting or joining bowel, since it allows you to identify the supplying vessels in the mesentery.

Probes and catheters

Place a probe or catheter in a track or duct that you wish to excise or preserve, as a marker. The technique is valuable during the excision of a thyroglossal fistula. On occasion it is a valuable help to insert a ureteric catheter before excising an extensive and adherent tumour nearby. You can then often preserve the ureter from inadvertent damage. If you need to resect a portion of it, you can take the appropriate steps to deal with the problem. If you have not marked it, you may be unaware of it and therefore unprepared for the consequences.

Dyes

Some surgeons inject a coloured dye, such as vital blue dye, into a complicated fistulous track as a marker. I have not found it very helpful because the dye tends to leak widely and stain all the tissues.

A valuable technique when operating on breast and some other cancers is to inject vital blue dye around the lesion. This is taken up by the lymphatics and carried to the nearest lymph nodes, which are labelled 'sentinel' since they stand guard over the lymphatic pathways of spread. If the local sentinel nodes are excised and shown to be free of malignant cells it is likely that more distant nodes are also free of growth (see Fig. 7.10).

Marker stitch

You may wish to come back to a structure later in the operation or at a subsequent operation. You may have unexpectedly found a small doubtful lesion in the bowel and wish to complete the intended procedure and come back to it. Place a black silk marker stitch close to it so it is easy to find. When performing Hartmann's operation for obstructive carcinoma of the rectosigmoid colon, you bring out a terminal colostomy and close off the rectum. You may intend to return after an interval and establish colorectal continuity but the closed rectal stump may be difficult to identify. Mark it with a black silk stitch.

Intraoperative ultrasound scanning

Small probes can be used to help in locating important structures and also to indicate the substance. The combination of ultrasound with Doppler analysis (duplex scanning) allows you to detect blood flow in vessels. The technique has increasing value and is likely to be more extensively used.

Flexibility

1. Do not invariably display structures from only one direction. From time to time look from other aspects, especially so if you are in difficulty or uncertain. If you are using tension or distortion of the tissues to facilitate the procedure, relax it from time to time and review the situation with the tissues returned to their normal state.
2. Do not be limited in your technique. Make use of the whole range of possible skills to carry out the procedure safely. For this reason see as many other surgeons, in different specialties – you may find you can adapt some of their techniques and instruments to your own practice.

Priorities

Worry about problems in the correct order. Do not become obsessed with one problem at the expense of other considerations. Do not concentrate on details at the expense of important principles. If you encounter difficulty do not obsessively continue along the path of your original decision; review the possibilities and decide if you should change your priorities. Good surgeons incorporate all their findings into their decisions.

REFERENCE

1. Henry AK. *Extensile exposure applied to limb surgery*. Edinburgh: E & S Livingstone; 1945.

Handling bleeding

Full discussion of prevention and control of bleeding demands a major textbook. In a monograph on basic techniques it is possible only to outline the practical management in the operating theatre. You should prepare yourself by studying the background science of bleeding and clotting.

HAEMORRHAGE

(G *haima* = blood + *rhegnynai* = to burst.)

Arteries bleed bright red blood in spurts when cut. They usually constrict and seal if they are transected, provided they are healthy. Because the aorta contains no muscle, it cannot contract when breached. Diseased, calcified arteries and those with side holes cannot contract efficiently.

Veins ooze dark blood. They can constrict – but do not trust them! Remember the peripheral valved veins bleed from distally – but if proximal valves are defective, they may bleed from proximal sources. Venous sinuses are held open – for example, intracranial sinuses do not constrict when they are breached.

Capillary bleeding stops following gentle compression – provided there is no clotting defect.

1. Primary haemorrhage occurs during operation or injury.
2. Reactionary bleeding results in the postoperative period when the blood pressure recovers, or straining raises venous pressure, dislodging respectively arterial and venous clots.
3. Secondary haemorrhage is the result of infection, with bacterial dissolution of occluding clots.

Key points

- Uncontrolled bleeding encourages hasty, ill-considered actions that prejudice surgical success.
- Anticipate and prevent bleeding by correcting anaemia and clotting defects.
- If bleeding is likely, ensure you have ordered adequate volumes of cross-matched blood.

PREVENTION

1. Study the anatomy so you can expose and control major vessels before you cut them.
2. When you encounter an important blood vessel that must be preserved, obtain control by placing across it a non-crushing clamp ready to be closed if necessary, or encircle it with flexible silicone rubber slings or tape (see Ch. 5).

Fig. 10.1 Doubly clamp and divide the vessel. Note that the curved haemostats are placed with their concave surfaces facing each other. This will facilitate the application of the ligatures beneath them.

3. If you wish to divide a major vessel, display it, pass two ligatures under it and tie them at a distance from each other and divide the vessel between them. Alternatively, apply haemostats on each side of the point of division, section the vessel, then ligate each cut end (Fig. 10.1). Do not apply the clamps too close together or the ligatures will be too near the cut ends and may slip off. Sometimes you can achieve sufficient space by applying three clamps, removing the middle one, and cutting through the space left by it (Fig. 10.2).

4. When tying very large arteries be prepared to place three artery forceps side by side and cut through the vessel leaving two forceps on the proximal stump.

Fig. 10.2 To create sufficient space between the clamps when a short segment only can be exposed, gently apply three clamps side by side and remove the middle one. This ensures that there is a sufficiently long stump presenting beyond the ligatures.

Tie a ligature under the deeper of the two forceps and remove it, then tie and tighten a second ligature before removing the second pair of forceps.

5. If an arterial stump continues to pulsate after ligation it may gradually roll off a ligature. The safest method of avoiding this is to apply a transfixion suture–ligature. Pass a needled thread through the artery and tie it to the short end, encircling half the circumference, then take a full turn round the vessel and tie a triple throw knot. The transfixion prevents the ligature from being displaced.

6. If you are operating on vascular tissues or organs, obtain control of the feeding vessels. You can sometimes apply non-crushing clamps across a soft structure such as kidney or liver, without damaging it, or encircle a portion with a tape that can be pulled sufficiently tight to constrict the vessels without injuring the organ. The classic method of controlling bleeding from the liver was described by the Australian-born Hogarth Pringle (1863–1941) from Glasgow Royal Infirmary in 1908; he compressed the hepatic artery and portal vein in the free edge of the lesser omentum between his fingers and thumb.

7. Be doubly careful when working in the depths, since any bleeding will rapidly create a pool, hiding the site. Take particular care not to injure large veins at sites where they are held open by surrounding structures, as in the pelvis.

8. Do not open large central veins such as the internal jugular vein unless you have good control. When the patient inspires, air may be sucked into the heart and cause frothing, with immediate circulatory failure.

9. When dissecting in vascular tissues, avoid mass exposure. Prefer to tackle small sections at a time, gaining complete control before proceeding to the next section.

AIDS

Elevation

1. If you can lower venous pressure in the area of operation, the veins and capillaries collapse. When vessels are cut, bleeding is minimal and usually stops without delay.

2. Limbs can often be raised above body level during operations.

3. The whole body may be tilted. Sideways tilt allows the limb on the opposite side to be raised. Head up or down tilt is a standard part of many operations. The distinguished surgeon Friedrich Trendelenburg of Leipzig (1844–1923) placed the patient head down when operating on varicose veins to avoid venous congestion in the leg veins. It can also be used when operating in the pelvis. 'Reverse Trendelenburg', or

head up, is a valuable position when operating on the head and neck, or in the upper abdomen.

4. At the end of the operation place the limb or patient into a natural relationship before closing the wound to reveal any bleeding when the usual venous pressure is restored. The part may then be raised in some cases to maintain a lowered venous pressure and avoid congestion during healing.

Fluid infiltration

1. This is an effective and often ignored method of reducing bleeding during operations on vascular tissues. Inject sterile physiological saline as you move the needle point, after initially aspirating the syringe to ensure the needle point is not in a large vessel. The fluid raises the tissue pressure and renders the tissues translucent.
2. In appropriate circumstances, as an extra aid, add adrenaline (epinephrine) 1:200 000 to produce local vasoconstriction.

Transillumination

1. If you are entering an area where there may be large blood vessels. You may be able to raise it and view the light through it, particularly if you have rendered it translucent by fluid infiltration. Alternatively, you may insert a mobile sterile light source behind it.
2. Do not forget, though, that if there is a large vein in a part that you have elevated under tension, it will empty and so not be visible. Gently relax it.

Tourniquet

1. This is a valuable method when carrying out delicate operations on the limbs.
2. It is contraindicated in the presence of ischaemia, venous thrombosis from vascular disease or trauma, if the soft tissues are injured or infected, or if there are bony fractures.
3. First empty the limb by elevating it for 2 minutes.
4. Encircle the proximal part with orthopaedic wool and apply a pneumatic tourniquet over this. Secure the tourniquet with a bandage to prevent it from slipping.
5. You may further exsanguinate the limb by applying an Esmarch bandage of thin, flat, elastic rubber, starting at the tips of the digits, with overlapping turns. Run it as a spiral as far as the tourniquet and secure the end (Fig. 10.3).
6. Inflate the tourniquet quickly to 50–70 mmHg above systolic blood pressure for the upper limb, and 90–100 mm above systolic arterial pressure for the lower limb. Now unwind the Esmarch bandage.

Fig. 10.3 Place a pneumatic cuff proximally round the limb while it is held vertically. Apply an Esmarch bandage from distal to proximal. Inflate the tourniquet and then remove the Esmarch bandage.

7. Record the time of tourniquet inflation and frequently check the pressure. It is conventional to limit continuous inflation to 1 hour for the arm and 1½ hours for the leg. Release the tourniquet for 30 minutes before reinflating it.
8. At the end of the procedure release the tourniquet so you can ensure that all the blood vessels are sealed, before you close the wound.

Technical aids (see also Ch. 2)

1. Diathermy is a well-established method of sealing vessels before dividing them, sealing and dividing them simultaneously, or sealing vessels already cut and bleeding. Bipolar diathermy has additional safety because current passes only between the tips of forceps in which the tissue is grasped, and this is coagulated. Ligasure™ compresses vessels, electrosurgically obliterates the lumen by melting the collagen and forming a seal so a knife can be triggered to transect the vessel.
2. Ultrasonic vibration produces intracellular cavitation, cellular disruption, tissue heating, coagulation, tissue welding, depending on the frequency and power. If a vessel up to 2 mm diameter is gently compressed and low-power ultrasound applied, it reliably welds and occludes the lumen. At higher power it has a disruptive cutting effect and coagulates the vessels.

167

3. Laser produces a coherent high-intensity beam that causes vaporization of the tissues. The wavelength and thus the tissue absorption is determined by the medium within which the radiation is generated, such as carbon dioxide, neodymium yttrium aluminium garnet (Nd:YAG), or argon. The heating associated with tissue vaporization produces tissue destruction with coagulation of the small blood vessels.

> **Key points**
>
> • Bleeding is better prevented than arrested.
> • Just before you make a cut into unknown tissue, are you confident there is no blood vessel within it?

CONTROL

1. Control generalized oozing with manual pressure, possibly expanded and extended with a gauze pack, or a metal retractor pressing on a pack. Sometimes you can push a pack under a wound edge to exert pressure.
2. Once bleeding has occurred, identify and isolate the vessels, pick them up and ligate them or seal them with diathermy current.
3. If your first clip catches the vessel with its tip alone, it may be difficult to apply a ligature that does not fall off. Do not risk it. Hold the first clip vertically while you apply a second clip beneath it across the vessel with its tip projecting. Then remove the first clip (Fig. 10.4). Make sure, though, that you do not tent the surrounding tissue, lifting a deeper structure into the jaws of the second clip and damaging it. Do not pick up surrounding tissue and ligate it together with the vessel. Your ligature does not directly contact and hold the vessel; arteries can retract, escape from the ligature and rebleed.
4. If you inadvertently divide a major vessel, control it initially with direct finger pressure or by compressing the supplying vessel until you have identified it. If you cannot identify the supplying vessel but you know it passes through a particular tissue, try applying a non-crushing clamp – such as sponge-holding forceps. Do not be hasty, you may wish to repair the vessel. Do not compound the problem by risking injury to other structures. If you can control it with pressure, wait 5 minutes timed by the clock. As you cautiously reduce and eventually release the compression you will be surprised and encouraged at how much less dramatic is the bleeding. Do not proceed until you have made sure that you have identified the vessel, assessed the likelihood of further bleeding and confirmed that you have not caused any damage.

Fig. 10.4 A If you have merely captured the tip of a bleeding vessel with your first haemostatic clip, gently lift it up while you place a second clip across it, with the tip projecting. Now remove the first clip and ligate the vessel. **B** Do not clamp and ligate tissue surrounding the vessel, which could then retract out of the ligature.

5. Prevent calamitous generalized bleeding from happening during a well-conducted operation by proceeding step by step, controlling any bleeding as it occurs. You then have only a single problem on which to concentrate at any time.
6. Tears of vascular organs such as the liver and spleen may sometimes be controlled with sutures but bleeding may continue behind the stitches. Superficial capsular tears are usually amenable to the application of gelatin sponge or microfibrillar collagen powder. Fibrinogen-rich cryoprecipitate can be applied to a bleeding area followed by thrombin, producing rapid clotting. Massive resection is sometimes indicated, or in the case of the spleen, removal of the whole organ; in this case it is important to give the patient polyvalent vaccine, and in the case of children prophylactic penicillin is usually given. These are problems for specialists, since bleeding can often be controlled by interventional radiology.

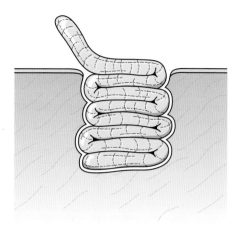

Fig. 10.5 Insert a long pack to control intracavity bleeding. Start in the depths and fold it back and forth like a jumping jack cracker. Either close the wound over the pack or bring out the end through the wound. Plan to remove it after 24–48 hours.

7. In some cases, simple packing suffices, as in the nose. Use a long pack; start in the depths and lay it back and forth like a jumping-jack cracker (Fig. 10.5). After 24–48 hours, return the patient to the operating theatre and, with the same preparations you used for the initial operation, cautiously remove the pack. Again, you may find that the bleeding has stopped.

> **Key points**
>
> - When faced with calamitous, life-threatening bleeding, never forget why you are here – to stop the bleeding!
> - Do not get carried away and perform any procedure that is not equally and urgently life-saving.

Intracavity bleeding

1. Unfortunately you do not have control of bleeding when a patient is admitted having sustained an injury or disease that has resulted in severe, life-threatening bleeding. A typical problem is bleeding within a closed cavity such as the abdomen and chest, since when you enter you may have no idea where the source lies. Tension builds up and eventually reduces the rate of bleeding.

2. When the cavity is opened, tension falls and bleeding starts with renewed force. Bleeding from a ruptured ectopic pregnancy, treated by open operation, requires prompt control. The introduction of laparoscopic methods allows the intraperitoneal pressure to be maintained and raised by insufflation, removing the need for urgency.

> **Key points**
>
> - When there is bleeding from an unknown source into a closed cavity, defer opening it until you have everything you need to deal with the problem – and have ensured that everything works.
> - As soon as you release the pressure, bleeding will start with renewed vigour.

3. Your hand may be forced when bleeding in the chest is causing serious cardiorespiratory distress. Have available a generous supply of large packs, two powerful suckers, large dishes in which to collect the large blood clots and long-handled artery forceps for clamping vessels in the depths. In addition, order vascular surgical instruments and sutures.

4. If you open the cavity and merely suck out the blood, you may exsanguinate the patient. Therefore, in the abdomen, open it swiftly and extensively, and insert packs into each quadrant, then pack the central area (Fig. 10.6). If necessary apply pressure until you have controlled the welling up of blood – but remember that compression squeezes out blood from the packs. Do nothing further except to scoop out loose blood and clots that will obscure your subsequent search for the origin of the bleeding, while the anaesthetist resuscitates the patient, restoring the blood volume.

5. If you have controlled bleeding and the patient's condition is improving, do not rush to 'do something', but carefully consider your options and tactics. Be willing to change your mind from your initial intentions. Ensure that you have all the help, equipment and instruments that you are likely to need.

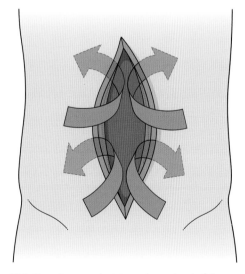

Fig. 10.6 Place large packs into each quadrant of the abdomen to control calamitous bleeding.

6. Arm your assistant with a sucker from which the guard has been removed. Peel back the edge of the central pack, compressing the part just behind the revealed area. If you see bleeding, isolate the smallest possible area and have your assistant maintain a clear field, using the sucker. Do not automatically clamp a vessel; you may wish to repair it. In many cases apply pressure just sufficient to control it with a finger, a pack or a gently applied non-crushing clamp.

7. As you control each area, continue to peel back the pack until you can remove it and start on the pack in the quadrant least likely to lie over the culprit. When this is finally removed, unpack the next most unlikely quadrant and so on, until, if all goes well, you are left with a final quadrant, having carefully checked and controlled all the others. Try to start at the highest point so that any bleeding will drain elsewhere. You may be pleasantly surprised to find that bleeding has diminished in the interval. Control it while you decide how best to deal with it.

Key points

- When you have stopped the bleeding Do Not Close Up!
- Wait while the anaesthetist restores the blood pressure and improves the patient's general condition.
- Have you removed all the blood that has collected? Stagnant blood makes an ideal culture medium.
- In your efforts to control the bleeding have you injured or imperilled any other structure?
- Once the bleeding is under control the situation is no longer urgent.

INTRACRANIAL BLEEDING

1. You may not rotate through a neurosurgical service but note that generalists see more head injuries than do neurosurgeons. Many of the consequences of head injury result from intracranial bleeding. Extradural haemorrhage may follow fracture of the temporal bone with tearing of the middle meningeal vessels; subdural haemorrhage may result from tearing of cerebral veins passing to the venous sinuses, often in elderly patients taking anticoagulants, following trivial injuries; intracerebral vessels rupture from distortion of the brain. Some patients develop small aneurysms, especially around the circle of Willis, which may rupture, causing a subarachnoid haemorrhage.

2. In addition to the primary brain damage, the patient may deteriorate as a result of secondary damage from ischaemia and oedema. Remember that the brain utilizes approximately 20% of the total body oxygen consumption, that ischaemia also produces cerebral oedema. The *basic surgical* action required is to maintain cerebral perfusion and oxygenation.

Key points

- Remember to maintain Airway, Breathing, Circulation.
- Be competent to administer oxygen at 12–15 L/min via a close-fitting face mask.

Handling drains

Abnormal accumulation of fluids – liquid, vapour or gas – may have deleterious effects from, for example, the space they occupy, pressure they exert, tracking within the tissues, susceptibility to infection or spread of existing infection, or absorption of toxic substances.

1. The value of most drains is hotly debated. As a trainee, follow the practice of the consultant who is responsible for the patients and watch the outcome so that you can draw your own conclusions about their value.
2. The use of drains can often be avoided by delaying operations if there is swelling that can be allowed to settle, by taking extra care over haemostasis, closure of vessels and ducts, and elevating parts to prevent the build-up of fluid swelling. In some cases the possible source of a collection can be brought to the surface.

3. In some circumstances drains are inserted as sentinels to warn of complicating blood or fluid discharge – but they are unreliable.
4. Drains can be used to bring together or keep together surfaces that would be separated by intervening fluids, such as air in the pleural cavity or oozing of blood from apposed raw surfaces.
5. In some cases the source can be brought to the surface where it can discharge and if the fluid to be drained is within a tube, a stoma can be formed.

> **Key points**
>
> - The value of drains is hotly debated.
> - Proponents claim they remove harmful fluids, monitor complications and do little harm.
> - Opponents claim they cause irritation, perpetuate discharge and offer an inward track for contamination.

CAUTION

1. In the absence of scientific knowledge or extensive personal experience, use drains where orthodox practice favours them.
2. As a trainee, follow the practice of your chief, but observe the results so you can develop your own views.
3. Use the softest and least irritant materials; ensure the drain does not press on damaged, delicate or vital structures, or suture lines.
4. If there is a main wound, prefer to bring the drain to the surface through a separate wound, to avoid prejudicing the healing of the main wound.

5. When possible make the track lead outwards and downwards to benefit from gravity drainage. When this is not possible and you must lead a drain down to a sump and suck it out, ensure that the drain tip reaches the lowest point, where fluid is likely to collect.

6. Whenever possible used a closed system to avoid the possibility of inward contamination.

TYPES

Packs and wicks

1. Gauze packs are sheets of sterile cotton gauze (Fig. 11.1), placed on a raw surface where discharge is expected to occur over a wide area, such as an abscess cavity, a laid-open superficial fistulous track, or as an initial treatment of an infected wound. It soaks up fluid most effectively if it is dry but some surgeons prefer it moistened with sterile isotonic saline solution or antiseptic solution. Unfortunately it needs to be changed frequently.

2. Gauze in contact with raw tissues soon adheres as it is invaded with fibrin threads. You can avoid this by soaking it in sterile liquid paraffin alone or emulsified with an antiseptic such as flavine. This destroys its ability to soak up fluid, which now tracks between the pack and the raw surface. As an alternative, first lay on a thin non-adherent net of tulle gras (F *tulle* = net + *gras* = fat), or a plastic substitute.

3. The absorbent pack may be overlaid with cotton wool so that it can be compressed with crepe bandage, a corset or by means of elastic adhesive strapping. Compression may reduce oozing and oedema. Since the cotton wool is intended to remain dry and elastic

Fig. 11.2 Gauze wick. This is a folded gauze sheet or ribbon, passed down a track to keep the track open.

to distribute the pressure evenly, make sure that it does not get soaked or it will form a hard cake; moreover, a completely soaked pack forms a moist channel for microorganisms from the exterior to the raw surface.

4. When the source of discharge cannot be brought to the surface, a wick of folded gauze or a gauze ribbon can be passed down to it (Fig. 11.2). It may block rather than hold open the channel. It is fully effective only until the gauze is soaked; thereafter it lies moistly and inertly in the channel. To avoid the wick becoming adherent to the tissues it may be passed through a thin-walled latex tube open at both ends (Fig. 11.3) – a so-called 'cigarette drain.' For very small tracks, twisted threads are sometimes inserted.

Sheet drains

1. A track may be kept open by inserting a sheet of latex rubber or plastic material (Fig. 11.4), which is often corrugated to create spaces. Alternatively, a Yeates drain (Fig. 11.5) comprises parallel plastic tubes. However, these are inert and fluid reaches the surface by gravity or *vis a tergo* (L = push from behind), where it must be soaked up by gauze packs. Fix them to prevent them from slipping into the wound by stitching them to the skin and also placing a large safety pin through the projecting portion.

2. Although these are not very effective, they are popular for the drainage of abscess cavities and to provide a track in case there is any subsequent discharge.

Fig. 11.1 Pack a wound with sterile cotton gauze. Make sure the pack is large enough to absorb the expected discharge. Cover it with dry gauze, which should remain dry and not become soaked.

Fig. 11.3 'Cigarette' drain. Pass a folded gauze sheet or ribbon through a thin-walled rubber tube open at both ends, where it acts as a wick.

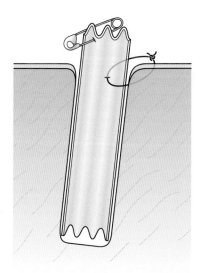

Fig. 11.4 A corrugated sheet drain of latex rubber or plastic material. It has been sutured in place and transfixed by a safety pin in the projecting portion.

Key point

- Packs, wicks and sheets are imperfect forms of drains but they are simple and usually serve their purpose in simple, localized infections after a track has developed spontaneously or been provided surgically.

Fig. 11.5 Yeates drain – a sheet formed of parallel tubes of plastic material.

Tube drains

1. These have the great advantage that they can lead away any content into a receptacle, such as a bag or other reservoir, thus forming a closed system, reducing the possibility of infection tracking back into the tissues. Tube drains usually have side as well as end holes (Fig. 11.6).
2. When fluid has entered the tube it may stagnate unless the tube is inserted upwards so it can drain by gravity. Fluid will flow only provided it is not viscous and only if the tube is sufficiently wide so that air can displace the fluid. If the tube is too narrow, the force of capillarity tends to retard the flow. However, fluid empties by *vis a tergo* if, for example, it is pushed out by a rise in intra-abdominal pressure. A limb may be compressed with a bandage to express any fluid into a drain – but compression of an infected area pushes the causative organisms into the bloodstream.
3. Usually the most effective method is to apply suction. Insert the tube so the tip lies at the lowest part where fluid is most likely to collect. The tube may be connected to a syringe fitted with a rubber bulb that is compressed before being attached, so that as it expands it exerts suction. A proprietary system uses a bottle that can be evacuated by a vacuum pump, then attached to the tube; the bottle cap incorporates an indicator to signal when the vacuum is lost.
4. The most versatile method is to apply suction directly from an electrically driven vacuum pump, incorporating a reservoir to collect any discharge

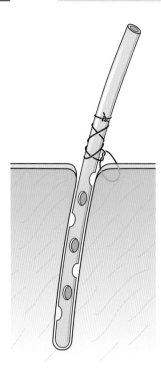

Fig. 11.6 A tube drain with multiple side holes, of silicone rubber or plastic material. Note how it is secured by tying the suture thread back and forth around it, then with a stitch through the skin that is loosely tied. The tube has not been transfixed and therefore will not leak.

Fig. 11.7 The Shirley wound drain incorporates a side tube guarded by a bacterial filter so that, when you apply suction to the main tube, sterile air can be drawn down to the drain tip, helping to prevent tissues from being sucked into the side holes and blocking them.

from the drain. The suction tends to drag tissue into the holes of the drain and block them, rendering the system ineffective. This can be partially overcome by using a pump that automatically and intermittently breaks the vacuum, allowing the pressure to rise to atmospheric – but the tissues may remain trapped in the holes.

The Shirley drain (Fig. 11.7) allows air to leak throughout, drawn in by the suction through a side tube protected by a bacterial filter. However, the most effective method is to use a sump drain (Fig. 11.8). Place a large tube with side holes at the bottom of a cavity so that any fluid will collect in it. Lying free within this is a suction tube which can take up the fluid but cannot be blocked by sucking in tissues.

5. The need for surgical creation of a path to the site of drainage has markedly diminished as methods of imaging have improved so that percutaneous aspiration and drainage can be accomplished, often using the Seldinger technique (Ch. 5). In some cases a pig-tail catheter can be passed into a cavity and the curl at the inner end acts as a retainer; alternatively, a Foley balloon catheter can be passed.

6. Normal fluids may be drained to monitor them. A classical example is a 'T-tube' inserted into a bile duct that does not necessarily drain bile unless the distal flow is blocked (see Fig. 4.12). When free flow is confirmed, the tube can be gently withdrawn. The hole closes spontaneously unless subsequent distal blockage develops.

SITES

Subcutaneous

1. Subcutaneous tissues vary in depth and vascularity in different individuals and in different parts of the body. Blood and reaction fluid collect, especially when the skin has been extensively undermined. Small collections can be drained using gauze wicks, corrugated sheet drains, or soft tubes with many side holes, connected to a gentle suction pump. They may

Fig. 11.8 Sump drain. The large outer tube creates a sump in which fluid collects. Lying freely in the bottom of the sump is a smaller tube attached to a sucker. Because the tissues are separated from the holes in the suction tube, they cannot be drawn in to block them.

be preferable to attempting to apply external pressure by means of cotton wool and crepe bandages in the hope of preventing fluid collecting.

2. Following extensive resection of, for example, the breast, the large potential space left following skin closure may accumulate oozed blood. Some patients develop a 'seroma' – a collection of serum. The best way of avoiding these complications is to encourage the skin to adhere to the base and obliterate the space. Compression is often ineffective and restricts respiration. Some surgeons insert multiple fine tubes with side holes connected to a suction pump or one of the many portable suction devices that are available such as a compressible bulb which exerts suction as it attempts to expand to its spherical shape.

3. In the presence of severe contamination or infection do not attempt to close the skin, vainly hoping that the drains will provide adequate removal of any discharge.

Subfascial and intramuscular

Do not trust drains in the presence of damaged muscle trapped beneath strong fascial coverings, since fluid collecting here raises the pressure, causing ischaemia, with the risk of infection from anaerobic organisms.

Extraperitoneal

After removing a source of intraperitoneal infection there is a risk of infection of the extraperitoneal tissues. Many surgeons close the peritoneum and leave a drain to its external surface, usually through a separate stab incision. An alternative is to leave the skin wound open and carry out delayed primary closure.

Intraperitoneal

1. This is the subject of bitter controversy. It was shown at the turn of the last century that a drain is usually sealed off within 6 hours. It is likely that the drain acts as a foreign body and that the discharge consists of reaction fluid in response to its presence. This may have resulted from the fact that the drains were formerly made of rubber; they are now usually made of Silastic, which is much less irritant.

2. On occasion intraperitoneal drains continue discharging fluid for prolonged periods if the amount of fluid generated prevents the surfaces coming together and sealing off. This occurs in ascites.

3. Although drains usually discharge fluid that is already present, the fiercest arguments centre around their ability to channel subsequent fluid collections to the surface and thus to signal a haemorrhage or the breakdown of an anastomosis with subsequent leakage into the peritoneal cavity. It is likely that all the criticisms and claims are correct in some circumstances.

Key points

- Use intraperitoneal drains, e.g. following open cholecystectomy, if it reassures you.
- Do not, though, allow the insertion of a drain to replace careful performance of the procedure.

4. Having inserted a drain, do not rely upon it to warn of a leak or a bleed if other features point to a complication.

5. Soft latex drains promote fibrosis and the formation of a track. Silicone elastomer, polyurethane and polyvinyl chloride are inert.

6. Insert drains through a small separate stab wound when possible. Take care to avoid major nerves and blood vessels in the abdominal wall. Keep the track straight by grasping the retracted peritoneum and posterior rectus sheath of the main wound on the side of the drain and draw them towards the opposite side. Now lift the whole abdominal wall upwards, clear of the viscera. Cut straight through the full thickness of the abdominal wall with a scalpel, taking care to cut the peritoneum under vision. Insert straight forceps through the stab wound and grasp the external end of the drain, to draw it out through the stab wound.

175

7. In some cases it is permissible to bring out the drain at one end of the main wound. If you do so, make sure you use separate stitches to secure the drain from those that close the wound. Eschew this, though, if infected material is likely to be discharged, for fear of contaminating the main wound.

8. Carefully place the inner end of the drain in the most dependent part where fluid is likely to accumulate but make sure there are no sharp ends pressing upon delicate structures.

9. Now insert a stitch through the skin and the drain, and tie it, leaving the ends long. If it is a sheet drain, place a large safety pin through it as an extra safety precaution to prevent if from dropping into the abdomen. If you are using a tube drain, insert the skin stitch, tie it loosely, then take a number of turns round the drain tube, back and forth, tying the ligature onto the drain without puncturing it. The tube drain can be connected in a closed manner, to a collecting bag.

10. Plan to remove intraperitoneal drains after 48 hours unless there is copious discharge. When a drain has been placed very deeply, it is sometimes removed by 'shortening it' a little each day.

Pleural cavity

1. Although liquid such as an effusion, pus or blood may be drained, an important function of chest drains is to remove air that has accumulated, has leaked following lung damage or enters through a breach in the thoracic wall. If the pleural space is occupied by air, the lung is compressed and collapses.

2. Introduce a tube through the chest wall, just above the upper border of a rib, in order to leave undamaged the neurovascular bundle that runs in a groove beneath the ribs (Fig. 11.9).

3. If there is a chest X-ray, examine it to determine the level of the diaphragm on each side, whether the lungs are collapsed, and whether there is any liquid in the pleural cavity. From the X-ray and by percussion and auscultation, decide where to insert the drain. You may decide the safest place is the fifth or sixth intercostal space in the anterior axillary line, the seventh or eighth space in the posterior axillary line or the second interspace anteriorly 3–5 cm from the lateral edge of the sternum.

4. You may insert the drain at the conclusion of a thoracic operation under general anaesthetic, in which case you can insert it under visual control. You may need to insert it in the ward with strict aseptic precautions, after infiltrating the skin and deeper tissues with local anaesthetic.

5. Make a 1–2 cm incision just above and parallel to the chosen rib and gradually deepen it to the pleura. Open the pleura and insert a finger to sweep it round 360° to ensure there is no adherent lung.

Fig. 11.9 Intrapleural drain with underwater seal. The tubular drain emerges through the chest wall, where it is secured by an encircling but not piercing stitch, which then catches the skin. Connect the tube to the vertical plastic tube passing through the bottle bung, the tip of which lies below the surface of sterile water in the bottom of the bottle. The short, angled tube allows air to escape from the bottle but can be attached to a source of suction.

6. Gently insert a chest drain after removing the trocar; there are side holes so make sure that they are all well inside the pleural cavity.

7. Insert strong, deep stitches on either side of, but not through, the tube, including the skin. Tie one loosely, leaving the ends long and then pass it back and forth around the tube, tying it after each encirclement, in the fashion of 'English lacing', to grip but not penetrate the tube, preventing it from being pulled out. Leave the other stitch untied and long, to be used to close the wound after withdrawing the tube.

8. Attach the outer end of the tube to sterile tubing that leads to an underwater seal bottle. The tubing is attached to a vertical plastic tube that pierces the bottle stopper and descends almost to the bottom of the bottle, which contains sterile water covering the lower end of the tube. There is another open tube that pierces the stopper and bends at a right angle so that organisms do not fall into it. If necessary this tube can be connected to a vacuum pump.

9. Place the bottle on the floor.

10. In the presence of a pneumothorax, if the intrapleural pressure rises above atmospheric, as the patient exhales, air is forced down the vertical tube and

bubbles out through the water. As the patient inhales, a short column of water is temporarily drawn up the vertical tube. During normal breathing the water level in the vertical tube oscillates, signalling that the tubes are patent and functioning correctly.

11. If liquid drains out of the chest it may be trapped in a dependent loop of tubing, damping the oscillation of the level in the vertical tube. Doubly clamp the tube emerging from the chest, disconnect the tubing distal to this, elevate the drain tube to allow the liquid to run into the bottle, then reconnect the tubes and take off the double clamps. Check that oscillation is now normal.

12. You can estimate the amount of liquid draining from the chest by marking the initial water level in the bottle and subsequently comparing the mark with the water level.

13. If air leaks rapidly into the pleural cavity, bubbling will continue in the bottle and the lung cannot re-expand. Check, and if necessary correct, any leakage around the chest drain. If not, connect the open tube emerging from the bottle to a vacuum pump set to maintain the pressure in the bottle at slightly below atmospheric pressure. This results in an increase in bubbling but eventually the lung will re-expand, seal against the parietal pleura, and the bubbling will cease. While you are applying suction do not expect to see any oscillation.

14. Intrapleural drains usually seal off and fail to function after 48 hours. You may now cut the stitch attaching the chest drain and withdraw it, tightening, as you do so, the loose stitch to seal off the hole. It is often valuable to apply suction as you gently withdraw the drain so that any last fluid collection is removed. Now tie the loose suture and apply a dressing.

ABSCESSES AND CYSTS

These are eminently suitable for drainage (see Ch. 12). After you have evacuated the contents the discharge will be small, but continue drainage to allow the cavity to shrink and become partly or completely obliterated. Depending on the site and size of the cavity, you may use open or closed drainage.

EXTERNAL FISTULAS

1. An external fistula opens on the body surface. Some produce little discharge and do not need to be drained. Others need to be excised or laid open and prevented from bridging over by applying packs.

2. Some fistulas, especially those carrying digestive juices from the gastrointestinal tract, may produce voluminous discharge which is usually intensely irritant to the skin or excoriating (L *ex* = off + *corium* = skin). The discharge can often be collected in a stoma bag. Cut an accurate hole in the karya gum backing to the stoma bag attachment ring, to fit closely around the discharge site. Clean and dry the skin around the stoma and apply the gum carefully to the skin. The stoma bag ring may have hooks to which you can attach an encircling belt. Clip on the stoma bag. This can be removed as necessary without disturbing the backing ring. In some cases the bag may be emptied from time to time, without removing it, through a tap at the bottom, or by removing and replacing a clip on a spout.

3. Less successful is a box that fits over the stoma, to which suction can be applied to maintain the seal. It works better in theory than in practice.

4. Occasionally you may be able to pass a Foley-type catheter into the fistulous track, gently inflate the catheter balloon to seal the passage, and allow the catheter to drain into a bag.

NEGATIVE PRESSURE WOUND HEALING

1. A number of devices have been developed to exert suction on open wounds. It is claimed that they act by removing discharged fluids and debris and encourage epithelialization.

2. The principle on which the devices work is that the wound is filled with a plastic foam shaped to the surface of the defect, in which is buried a tube connected to a vacuum pump. Alternatively the suction tube may be wrapped in gauze. Over the area a plastic sheet is laid and sealed round the edge to the skin with adhesive (Fig. 11.10).

Fig. 11.10 Negative pressure wound healing. The wound is filled with plastic foam shaped to fully occupy it. A tube is buried within the foam. The area is now sealed with plastic film which is stuck to the surrounding skin with adhesive. The tube is connected to a suction pump.

3. Suction of about 100–130 mmHg is applied by a suction pump.
4. Wound exudate is removed and possibly bacteria and loose slough. Various claims are made such as oedema is reduced, blood flow is increased, phagocytes and fibroblasts are promoted, and growth factors are increased. A wide variety of conditions have been treated using the method including diabetic foot.[1] Improved healing is claimed, although the Cochrane Reports have not identified any clear advantage.

REFERENCE

1. Armstrong DG, Lavery LA. Negative pressure wound therapy after partial diabetic foot amputation: A multi-centre, randomized controlled trial. *Lancet* 2005;366:1704–1710.

Chapter | **12** |

Handling infection

Infection (L *in* = into + *facere* = to make) strictly signifies disease spread through the air, while both contamination and contagion (L *con* = together + *tangere* = to touch) indicate transmission by direct contact. Sepsis (G = decay) usually implies the invasion of pathogenic bacteria or their toxins into the bloodstream or tissues.

PRINCIPLES

1. The capacity of microorganisms to cause infection depends on the balance between the virulence and numbers of the organisms on the one hand, and the health, vigour and nutritional state of the tissues on the other hand. It is increasingly recognized that local lack of tissue oxygen results in deprived and inactive phagocytes.[1] Another recently identified influence is the ability of communities of microorganisms to adhere and develop a polymeric matrix biofilm, impairing the efficiency of antibacterial efforts, particularly in elderly and immunocompromised patients.

2. While we should hope to operate on patients who are uninfected and clean, many of our patients require operation specifically because they are already infected.

3. It is essential that we employ our expertise as physicians to keep or raise the patient's condition to the best attainable state before operation, correcting fluid, electrolyte and nutritional status, recognizing and alleviating the effects of old age and obesity, and treating co-morbidity, including organ failure, compromised immunity, diabetes and drug addiction. Expertly performed surgery is useless if it is performed inappropriately, or on an ill-prepared patient.

4. Wounds are often classified in order to help predict the risks of subsequent infection:
   Clean wounds are typically elective, non-traumatic, technically perfect and primarily closed.
   Clean contaminated wounds include emergencies with minimal spillage such as appendicectomy in the absence of perforation.
   Contaminated encompasses non-purulent inflammation or spillage of gut, biliary, urinary or other fluids. Other conditions are those resulting from a major technical failure, penetrating trauma of less than 4 hours and chronic open wounds.
   Dirty wounds result from pus formation, gross perforation of gut, biliary or urinary tract and penetrating trauma more than 4 hours old.

INFECTIONS

Cellulitis

Cellulitis is a diffuse, spreading infection.

1. The virulent strains of *Streptococcus pyogenes* spread by causing fibrinolysis and pass up the lymphatic vessels and directly into the bloodstream.
2. Cellulitis within the dermis is called erysipelas (G *erythros* = red + *pella* = skin).
3. In cellulitis caused sometimes by group A *Streptococcus* alone, sometimes by synergistic (G *syn* = together + *ergon* = work) organisms including MRSA (meticillin-resistant *Staphylococcus aureus*) and *Clostridium perfringens*, toxins are released that result in destruction of soft tissues. Different sites acquired different names but it is now usually called *necrotizing fasciitis*.
4. The exotoxins of *Clostridium difficile* produce inflammation and mucosal cell necrosis in the gut, with severe diarrhoea as a result of changes in intestinal flora usually following prolonged courses of broad-spectrum antibiotics.

Abscess

An abscess (L *abs* = from + *cedere* = to go) is an enclosed cavity filled with necrotic material and the products of liquefaction, consisting mainly of dead phagocytes, which form pus (G *pyon* = L *pus*).

1. If an abscess forms near a surface, it may 'point', spontaneously rupture, and discharge to the body surface or to an internal space such as the peritoneal cavity, or into a hollow viscus such as the bowel. At first the swelling becomes reddened, hot and tender (classically described in Latin as *tumor, rubor, calor, dolor*). The rise in pressure empties the overlying blood vessels so that the centre becomes white, then darkens as it undergoes necrosis. At the body surface you can detect a point of maximal tenderness and softening, and elicit fluctuation in a larger abscess.
2. A boil (OE *byl* = an inflamed swelling) is an infection of a hair follicle, usually from *Staphylococcus aureus*, and may develop into a small abscess. It usually discharges or subsides spontaneously (a 'blind' boil).

SIRS AND SEPSIS

1. The clinical condition of systemic inflammatory response syndrome (SIRS) has become recognized to represent features common to a number of conditions.
2. SIRS is considered to be present if two or more of the following are present:

Heart rate >90/min
Temperature <36°C or >38°C
Respirations >20/min or blood P_aCO_2 <4.3 kPa
WBC <4000/mm³ or >12 000/mm³ or with more than 10% immature forms.
3. The syndrome usually results from trauma, burns, pancreatitis and some other conditions.
4. If it results from infection it is defined as sepsis.

VIRAL TRANSMISSION

1. The most important viruses are human immunodeficiency virus (HIV), hepatitis B virus (HBV) and hepatitis C virus (HCV).
2. You can protect yourself and your colleagues by ensuring that you do not risk coming into contact with human blood or blood products and human natural secretions. Make sure you do not sustain, or cause anyone in the team to sustain, skin damage. Be especially careful of needle-stick injuries and injuries with other sharp instruments. Never pass them from hand to hand; always place them in a dish whenever they are not being used or when they are being passed from one person to another.
3. Although homosexual males, intravenous drug users and haemophiliacs treated before 1985 are high risk, make your precautions universal. It is dangerous to assume that people who do not fall into the high-risk categories are free of infection.

UNIVERSAL PRECAUTIONS

These rules were developed, in addition to standard precautions, in response to the outbreak of acquired immune deficiency syndrome (AIDS) in the 1980s.

1. The title is often quoted with the assumption that the precautions are well understood. Most rules are discretionary; 'universal' signifies 'without exception'.
2. All patients with whom you come into contact must be assumed to be possible carriers of pathogens in certain body fluids, such as blood, semen and vaginal secretions, and peritoneal, pleural, pericardial, synovial and amniotic fluids.
3. Wash hands before and after each medical procedure, or apply non-aqueous cleaner.
4. Wear protective gloves when at risk of coming into contact with potentially pathogenic fluids.
5. Wear a protective gown, face mask and eye covers if there is danger of body fluid splashing onto you.
6. Safely dispose of contaminated sharp instruments including needles.
7. Safely dispose of contaminated protective equipment.
8. Universal precautions need not be applied to nasal fluids, saliva, sputum, vomitus, urine or faeces.

Key point

- Do not ignore universal precautions in emergency situations.

TRAUMA

Traumatized tissues are often contaminated and resulting loss of vitality means that sepsis may develop.

1. Before operation on a patient with an injury, carefully assess and investigate the injuries to soft tissue, skin, bones and joints, blood vessels and nerves and the presence of foreign bodies. This allows you to plan your strategy ahead and to order any equipment and back-up that you will need.
2. Every surgical operation is traumatic. Do not compound it by handling the tissues roughly. Injured tissues have increased susceptibility to infection as a result of contamination.
3. Under suitable anaesthetic induction, open and explore the wound one layer at a time. Gently remove all dead tissue, ensuring that all remaining tissue is clean and viable. Viable muscle should bleed when cut, contract when pinched. Dead muscle appears pale and homogeneous, is friable and does not contract when pinched. Seek and remove all fragments.
4. Make use of lavage with sterile physiological saline to wash out fragments of foreign material.
5. It is particularly dangerous to introduce, or fail to remove, microorganisms that require little or no oxygen for their metabolism within damaged, dead or ischaemic tissues.
6. Battle injuries and traffic accidents cause risk of severe infections. Penetrating injuries allow organisms to be carried deeply. High-velocity missiles, especially bullets fired from high-velocity rifles and shrapnel scattered from an explosion, are particularly dangerous. They carry in clothing and other foreign material. If the kinetic energy of the missile is rapidly dissipated in the tissues, it acts like an explosive, disrupting the cells. Anaerobic organisms flourish in the resulting dead tissue. For this reason it is essential to remove all dead tissue and foreign material, and expose the retained healthy tissue to the air.

Key points

- Systemically administered antibiotics cannot reach dead or ischaemic tissues.
- Do not close a wound if you are uncertain if it is recent, healthy, with no foreign material and tension-free.
- In case of doubt employ delayed primary closure (see Ch. 6).

PREOPERATIVE

1. We all have microorganisms constantly with us on our skin, in our noses, mouths, and gut and we may become infected as a result of contact with other people or infected material, especially if we have exposed cuts or injuries or have diminished resistance.
2. Many of the operations surgeons perform are for the treatment of existing infection. Patients submitting themselves to operation often carry organisms that could be carried to the site of operation. Many organisms are harmless in one site, as in the gut, but are harmful elsewhere.
3. Hospitals are reservoirs of nosocomial infection (G nosos = sickness + komeien = to tend; hospital sickness) from organisms often resistant to antibiotics. Although they may be harboured in instruments, dressings and bedding, many studies have demonstrated that transmission of the majority of infections is by personal contact. This can occur between patients, or via nurses and doctors, especially if effective hand-washing is neglected between encounters.
4. Consider the need for prophylactic or peroperative antibiotics, especially for someone at increased risk, including patients with a prosthesis such as a heart valve replacement.

OPERATING ROUTINES

1. Before 'scrubbing up', check your hands for cuts, abrasions and ulceration. If you find any, apply a waterproof adhesive dressing.
2. During procedures placing you at risk, wear a long apron, an impervious gown, eye shields and double gloves. If your gloves are damaged, change them.
3. Keep all sharp instruments in separate dishes. Never pass them by hand.
4. Avoid spilling blood as far as possible by sealing vessels before you divide them.
5. To reduce the risk of spreading infection on surgeons' gloves during the operation, Sir Arbuthnot Lane (1869–1943) successfully popularized 'no touch' techniques. All the procedures were carried out using instruments. A modification of the technique is continued in minimal access procedures.
6. If you sustain a needle-stick injury, encourage bleeding, wash your hands, and put on fresh gloves as soon as you can. Afterwards report it to the Occupational Health Officer.
7. As a routine, at the end of every operation check your hands for any injuries you may not have noticed while concentrating on the procedure.

OPERATION

1. In the past the skin was assiduously shaved, washed and prepared with sterilizing applications before operation. Shaving is now avoided because of the resultant damage to the skin; if necessary, the hairs are clipped short, using a clipper with a disposable head.

2 Before making the incision, clean the skin with an antiseptic solution such as 2% iodine in 50% ethanol or 0.5% chlorhexidine in 70% ethanol. Drape the area with sterile towels, usually proprietary disposable sheets, to isolate the operation site. Some towels cover a wide area and have a central hole through which you make the approach. If you apply several towels, fix them together with towel clips. Alternatively, or in addition, you may apply a sterile, transparent, adhesive sheet through which you make the incision.

3. You may be operating to deal with an existing infection, or in an area where there are organisms present that are harmless here but would be dangerous if they spread elsewhere. In both cases take every possible precaution to avoid disseminating the organisms. Pack off tissues outside the immediate area of the operation. Remove immediately, or isolate, contaminated material. Keep all the instruments used in the contaminated area in a special container, to be discarded as soon as the 'dirty' part of the operation is completed. If it is essential for you to handle contaminated or potentially contaminated material and tissues to assess them, or as part of the procedure, discard your gloves and replace them with sterile ones before completing the operation. Similarly discard and replace soiled drapes.

4. If you encounter infection, always take a specimen or swab for culture and tests of sensitivity to antibiotics.

5. At the end of the operation the whole area should be clean and viable.

6. Should you close the wound?

7. Be willing to lightly pack the wound and wait until it is clean, healthy, free of discharge and then close it, if necessary by applying a skin graft.

8. If you have closed the wound, or if you are dealing with a closed injury, frequently and carefully watch to exclude swelling and tissue tension. This may be most obvious in a limb. If necessary carry out debridement (F = unbridle – the original meaning was to cut away constricting bands; only later was it extended to mean excision of dead tissue). Incise the skin and deep tissues longitudinally to release the tension. Lay in sterile gauze and replace it at intervals until the wound is suitable for closure or grafting.

9. Mesothelial-lined cavities such as the peritoneal space may be contaminated, as when large bowel is breached surgically, by trauma or disease, releasing organisms within the peritoneum. It may be necessary to create an artificial opening of the colon onto the abdominal wall – a colostomy. Remove every trace of colonic content from the peritoneal cavity with warm, sterile, physiological saline. Once it is free of contamination, the peritoneum is usually well able to resist infection. However, the superficial part of the wound is much more susceptible. You should either drain the superficial layers or leave them open.

10. The precepts of Kocher, Halsted and Cushing of gentleness, haemostasis and perfect tissue apposition did not specifically include oxygenation. Ischaemia (G *ischein* = to restrain + *haima* = blood) was well recognized but tissue anoxia (G *an* = not + oxygen + *ia* = indicating a pathological condition) is not always clinically detectable.

BLEEDING

Stagnant blood provides an ideal culture medium for micro-organisms. The incidence of wound infection is increased after operations in which excessive bleeding has occurred. Make every effort to leave the operative field completely dry, removing all spilled blood, and guard against continuing or recurring bleeding when the procedure is completed.

SURGICAL SITE INFECTION

The incidence of infection at the site of operation is related to bacterial factors, surgical technique and the patient.

1. Bacterial factors include the type: *Staphylococcus aureus* and *Escherichia coli* are commonly involved but other organisms including fungi may be causative. Bacteria in one site may be harmless for example within the gut, but be pathological elsewhere.

2. Surgical factors include whether the wound is clean or dirty, the perfection of operating technique, operating time, presence of necrosis and the presence of foreign materials or prostheses.

3. The patient's age, immune status and nutritional state affect resistance and this is reduced in obesity, diabetes, malignancy, co-morbidity and as a result of smoking.

4. Surgical site infections contribute significantly to the approximately 9% of hospital-acquired infections within National Health Service Trusts.[2] The Nosocomial (hospital-related) Infection National Surveillance Scheme, started in 1996, revealed that 50–70% of surgical site infections (SSIs) occurred post-discharge from hospital.

5. The incidence of surgical site infections is dependent on wound type, operation class, use of drainage, the operating surgeon and American Society for Anesthesiologists (ASA) category: I, healthy; II, mild systemic disease; III, severe systemic disease; IV, severe disease a constant threat to life; V, moribund, unlikely to survive 24 hours. To enable comparison of outcomes, the Health Protection Agency Surgical Site Infection Surveillance Service (SSISS) collects results from mandatory surveillance according to the type of operation and issues comparative tables.[3]

TREATING INFECTIONS

Cellulitis

1. Early, adequate, treatment with a well-chosen antibiotic is usually the most important step in the management of many forms of cellulitis.

2. Obtain a specimen for culture and immediately deliver it to the microbiologist, at the same time taking advice on the antibiotic most likely to be effective.

3. Operative treatment is urgently required if there is necrosis, especially in the case of necrotizing fasciitis. All the necrotic tissue must be excised, leaving only healthy tissue.

4. If there is an underlying cause for the cellulitis, you must deal with this.

Abscess

1. One of the principal functions of surgeons was traditionally to 'let out the pus'. Access to imaging methods has replaced many operative procedures. Simple ultrasonic viewing of the collection of pus facilitates the insertion of a drain following injection of local anaesthetic. Small abscesses can be drained through a needle, or catheter carried on a needle or using Seldinger's technique (see Ch. 5). Larger abscesses may demand a small incision to accommodate a formal drain (see Ch. 11).

2. Be sure that there is no continuing cause for the abscess or simple drainage will not suffice.

3. Local anaesthesia is less effective in the presence of inflammation but in many localized situations it spares the patient the need of a general anaesthetic. If

you intend to employ it, raise an intracutaneous bleb in adjacent uninflamed skin and slowly and gently inject ahead of the needle until you have reached the pinnacle of the abscess. If you are impatient and inject under pressure, raising the tissue tension, you will cause pain. If you do not wait long enough for the anaesthetic to take effect, you have wasted your time and will hurt the patient. Never incorporate adrenaline (epinephrine) with the local anaesthetic or you may cause extensive necrosis.

In the case of a finger pulp infection, if you create a ring block at the base of the finger, you must avoid at all costs creating a constricting ring of swelling; if you do, the whole finger may undergo necrosis. Inject only within the web space where the volume of fluid will not have any constricting effect.

> **Key points**
>
> - Many abscesses can be drained using a needle and syringe with a three-way tap to empty the syringe.
> - Deep abscesses are often best drained using a catheter introduced under imaging control.

4. Incise an abscess at the point of greatest tenderness, or on the pinnacle of the swelling. Obtain a swab for culture and determination of antibiotic sensitivity. Clean out the contents, taking a specimen for culture. If you have any doubts about the aetiology, excise a portion of the edge for histological examination.

5. Empty the contents not by squeezing, which will introduce organisms into the bloodstream, but with a scoop, or by washing out with fluid from a syringe. Squeezing of infected lesions is particularly deprecated on the face around the nose and upper lip. Organisms will drain by the anterior facial vein into the cavernous venous sinus and may cause septic thrombosis.

6. Unless this is an obviously small local abscess, insert a finger or an instrument to explore the interior for loculations (L *loculus* = diminutive of locus = place) or track. Collar-stud abscess is notorious in the neck when a diseased lymph node undergoes necrosis and liquefaction; the resulting pus then tracks through a hole in the deep fascia to form a subcutaneous abscess. Tuberculous cervical lymph node is a well-known cause. An infected branchial cyst may also create a collar-stud abscess.

7. An abscess near the anus may develop from infected anal gland, presenting close to the anal margin. An ischiorectal abscess, developing higher up, usually presents laterally and further away. You may be able to feel and open up loculi and detect an upward extension with a finger in the abscess cavity. Do not attempt to probe it in search of an internal opening.

It is usual to pack the wound to prevent it from healing over until the base has filled up. If the skin is allowed to close over, an abscess may reform.

8. An intra-abdominal abscess usually results from localized disease that has been limited from spreading by adhesion of surrounding structures. A typical condition is appendix abscess. When the appendix becomes inflamed, surrounding structures usually adhere and form an appendix mass. If the appendix then ruptures, it does so into a constrained cavity. You need to be very cautious and gentle in approaching the mass for fear of releasing the contents into the general peritoneal cavity, or of damaging any of the inflamed, fragile viscera forming part of the wall of the mass. Be content to drain the abscess unless the appendix is easily found within the cavity and can be removed without disturbing the other structures.

9. Some other abscesses within the abdomen, which have an underlying cause, may not settle after you drain them. Leakage from a viscus may continue and a track will form to the surface, creating a fistula (see Ch. 4).

10. Having emptied the abscess you need to maintain drainage. A wick or ribbon of gauze is sometimes inserted into a small abscess. Very often this merely acts as a plug. The drain should keep the wound open until the cavity is completely empty, and in some cases until it has had time to shrink and fill up with granulation tissue. Therefore, prefer soft latex corrugated sheet, usually held by a single stitch. If the cavity is deep, insert a safety pin into the projecting portion as an extra precaution so that it cannot fall into the cavity (see Ch. 11).

11. If possible arrange that the drainage hole will be dependent so that the cavity will drain by gravity. This may be difficult in the breast. It is rarely necessary to make a second incision from the undersurface of the breast to drain a high, deeply placed abscess.

REFERENCES

1. Allen DB, Maguire JJ, Mahdavian M, et al. Wound hypoxia and acidosis limit neutrophil bacterial killing mechanisms. *Arch Surg.* 1997;132:991–996.

2. National Audit Office. *The management and control of hospital-acquired infection in acute NHS Trusts in England.* London: Her Majesty's Stationery Office; 2000.

3. Health Protection Agency, Surgical Site Infection Surveillance Service (SSISS): Online. http://www.hpa.org.uk; (click on Topics A–Z).

Chapter | **13** |

Handling minimal access surgery

Minimal access procedures comprise those internal manipulations that can be performed without the need for extensive exposure to reach the target tissue. Traditionally, surgeons were encouraged to employ generous incisions, allowing careful exploration and ample access, by the adage that 'wounds heal from the sides, not from the ends'. The need for wide exposure has been markedly reduced by the development of improved imaging methods and technical advances; these have often been achieved by incremental improvements in what were originally unpromising innovations.

Key points

- As new approaches and techniques are developed in one area they are seized upon and utilized in others – skills are transferable!
- Anticipate soundly based advances and be prepared to acquire new skills that are often needed to exploit demonstrable patient benefits.

Examples

1. Conventional open procedures performed through the smallest possible incisions, prefixed 'mini-', such as laparotomy, cholecystectomy, appendicectomy. Special long-handled but conventional instruments may be used.
2. Radiological, magnetic resonance, ultrasound and other methods of imaging allow interventions using needles and cannulas. Many of them depend on developments of Seldinger's technique (see Ch. 5) by means of which access can be gained into blood vessels, ducts, natural, pathological and created spaces. In neurosurgery carefully targeted instruments may be passed through burr holes to biopsy, or destroy by ultrasonic, electrosurgical or other means, special tissues or tumours. A frame can be attached to the skull to hold the instrument but this has largely been replaced by computer-generated targeting.
3. Endoscopy is generally recognized to have developed from fibreoptics in rigid or flexible guided instruments passed through natural ducts with any procedures performed along the line of sight or aided by imaging techniques. Endoscopic retrograde choledocho-pancreatography allows visualization which can be augmented by imaging for diagnostic and therapeutic procedures.
4. 'Minimal access surgery' generally implies procedures carried out in the main by surgeons as opposed to radiologists and endoscopists. It depends upon simultaneous developments in illumination, visualization, instruments – and more importantly, the willingness of pioneers to acquire new, complex skills that often require natural movements to be reversed. A major step forward was the realization

that instruments that were previously inserted along the line of sight could often be inserted through separate ports allowing them to be viewed with better depth perception. It has succeeded in spite of other deficiencies – two-dimensional viewing on a screen with loss of binocular vision, haptic loss (the sense of touch) with reduced appreciation of force and torque transmitted to the tissues, and reversal of some natural manipulative functions. Wherever a cavity exists, even though it is potential only, it may be possible to expand it with carbon dioxide, saline, or initially with a balloon, to allow the insertion through separate portals of a combined light and camera, and instruments to perform a rapidly increasing variety of surgical procedures. In some centres space is created within the abdomen by lifting the abdominal wall instead of inflating it with gas.

5. Robotic surgery is a further demonstration that once a technique has been shown to be practicable, small incremental improvements are developed that make it likely to become widely available. It offers the advantage that the operator's surgical movements feel natural, hand tremor is eliminated, binocular vision is available and haptic sensation is promised. In the past the initial high cost of all electronically controlled instruments has rapidly fallen as manufacturers compete for the market and demand increases as users compete to exploit the newly available technical possibilities. It is likely that this facility will develop and be widely available.

Laparoscopy

ACCESS

This is not a new concept. For many years abdominal surgeons routinely employed a rigid sigmoidoscope inserted through a small stab incision, inflating the abdomen using the hand pump. Limited areas could be visualized and biopsies removed along the line of sight. The German physician Kalk was the first to use separate access points for needles inserted across the line of sight to obtain liver biopsies. The gynaecologist Kurt Semm of Kiel is considered the father of modern laparoscopy. Laparoscopy (G *lapara* = flank or loins from *laparos* = soft, loose + *skopein* = to view) is normally carried out under general anaesthesia.

1. Obtain consent for the procedure to be converted to an open operation if necessary.
2. Make sure the bladder is empty; if necessary, pass a catheter.
3. If the stomach is distended, pass a nasogastric tube.
4. Carefully palpate the relaxed abdomen to identify any masses and locate the sacral promontory. Percuss the abdomen to detect the lower level of liver dullness.

Two methods have been developed to allow safe penetration of the abdominal wall without damage to intra-abdominal viscera or major blood vessels.

Closed pneumoperitoneum

This was initially popular.

1. Make a small sub-umbilical incision down to but not through, the peritoneum. Pick up the abdominal wall and gently insert the Veress needle (Fig. 13.1). As the point penetrates the peritoneum, a spring-loaded, round-ended obturator projects, pushing away any underlying structure.

> **Key point**
>
> • Listen for, and feel for, the click as the Veress needle obturator extends.

2. Check your confidence in the safety of peritoneal puncture by opening the tap on the Veress needle and place a drop of sterile saline on the Luer connection. The drop should be drawn into the needle when the patient inhales. Gently inject 10 mL saline through the needle, then try to aspirate it; if you can, the needle tip must be in a closed space. Switch on the insufflator (L *in* + *sufflare* = to blow) with a gas flow of 1 litre/min and check the pressure, which should not exceed 8 mmHg. Confirm that liver dullness has been lost.
3. If all is well, cautiously inflate the abdomen with 3–5 litres carbon dioxide, provided the abdomen is evenly distended and pressure is 10–15 mmHg. Now withdraw the Veress needle and enlarge the incision down to the peritoneum.
4. Insert the trocar with its cannula, which has a flap or trumpet valve to prevent gas leakage (Fig. 13.2). Hold the trocar and cannula in the palm of the hand with index finger extended to limit the extent

Fig. 13.1 A Veress needle. **A** The needle is just about to pierce the inner lining of the cavity. **B** As soon as the needle has entered the cavity, the round-ended, spring-loaded obturator projects, pushing away any structure that might be punctured by the sharp needle and exposing the gas inlet.

2. Insert a finger and sweep it in a full circle to confirm that you have reached the peritoneal cavity and that there are no adherent viscera. Grasp the edges of the incision and insert two strong, 0 monofilament polyamide or polypropylene stitches taking a good bite of the linea alba and peritoneum, one above the centre of the incision, one below the centre. Capture the untied ends in forceps. Alternatively, insert a single stitch as a purse-string, encircling the centre of the incision and capture the untied ends.

3. Insert a 10 mm diameter Hassan cannula (Fig. 13.3), which has a blunt obturator and a conically shaped neck intended to block the entrance hole and stop leakage; either a standard cannula with a blunt obturator or a standard cannula with the trocar removed. Some cannulas have an encircling inflatable balloon to fit just beneath the peritoneum, to prevent leakage of gas from the abdomen.

4. Draw the stitch or stitches tight and tie them around the cannula projections and loop them over the gas inlet. Do not knot the threads but clip them, so you can use them to close the incision at the end of the procedure.

5. Gently ensure that the cannula moves freely. If all is well, connect the gas inlet to the insufflator, which is set to deliver carbon dioxide at 1 litre/min and against a pressure not exceeding 12–15 mmHg.

Fig. 13.2 A The cannula has the sharp trocar in place. **B** The head of the trocar sits in the palm of your hand and your index finger extends along the shaft of the cannula to prevent too deep penetration. Aim the trocar towards the anus, i.e. below the previously identified sacral promontory using a gentle twisting motion.

of penetration, inserting it with a twisting motion, directing the tip below the previously identified sacral promontory, pointing towards the anus. You can meanwhile distend the lower abdomen by gently compressing the upper abdomen. As the trocar pierces the peritoneum, a spring-loaded collar may project, extending beyond the sharp tip of the trocar. Listen for the click.

5. Withdraw the trocar and replace it with the combined light carrier, telescope and camera, attached to the light source and television monitor. View the interior to check that there has been no damage.

Open pneumoperitoneum

This is now generally preferred.

1. Make a 1.5–2 cm incision, either vertical just below the umbilicus, or transversely sub-umbilical. Carry it down to the linea alba, identified by the white fibres after which it is named (L *albus* = white). Other sites may be more appropriate if there are nearby scars on the abdomen. Incise the linea alba leaving the peritoneum intact, to be tented and incised separately, or grasp and lift the linea alba on each side with strong forceps while you cut through it and proceed to open the peritoneum.

Fig. 13.3 Hassan cannula. The coned neck blocks the entrance hole. The cannula is usually held in place by deep stitches on each side, tied over projecting shoulders to prevent displacement of the cannula. Some models have a screw shape and remain in place even without retaining stitches. The insufflator, camera and lighting systems are connected. Subsequent ports are inserted while you watch their entrance from within, to avoid damage to internal structures.

TECHNICAL ASPECTS

1. Space has been created with carbon dioxide gas from the insufflator, delivered at a predetermined rate to the required volume, up to a preset pressure, sounding an alarm if this is exceeded. For some procedures, carried out extraperitoneally, a space can be developed by inserting a balloon without breaching the peritoneum. One technique does not require pneumoperitoneum; the abdominal wall is lifted from the viscera with a coat-hanger-like instrument.

2. Introduce the combined light and miniature camera and watch the entry sites on the television monitor as you introduce further valved cannulas through which various instruments can be freely introduced and withdrawn. Identify and avoid large vessels, particularly the inferior epigastric blood vessels. Because instruments can then be manoeuvred across, rather than along the line of sight, their spatial relationships with the target structure can be accurately judged. Site these ports in order to provide the most advantageous approach and available space for instruments. There are standardized port sites for many operations but take into consideration the patient's build and the presence of scars.

3. A single fixed camera entry point limits the view of structures, usually to one aspect and, at present, a two-dimensional view on the monitor screen. A second monitor provides a view for the assistant controlling the camera and for the scrub nurse.

4. The instruments are long-handled and slide in and out through the fixed entry portal in the abdominal wall, which forms the fulcrum. As the instruments are withdrawn and advanced, the relationship is changed between the inner and outer portions, so changing the amount of movement produced at the tip of the instrument resulting from a standard movement of the handle (Fig. 13.4). The tip can be moved anywhere within a cone whose apex is at the body wall.

Fig. 13.4 The effect of withdrawing and advancing an instrument through the access port on the volume of accessible space. The effect also alters the inverse relation between hand movements and movements at the instrument tip. If the instrument is almost fully inserted a small hand movement produces an extensive movement of the instrument tip, and vice versa. This demonstrates the importance of carefully placing the entry portal to achieve a correct balance between internal and external length of operating instrument.

> **Key points**
>
> - When siting the entrance port, carefully consider the required range of movement of the instrument tips in relation to your hand movements.
> - Ports sited too close to the target structure commit you to wide hand movements; sited too far away they commit you to making very limited hand movements and exaggerated tip movements.

5. Retractors, suckers, irrigators, forceps clip applicators, staple applicators and other newly developed instruments are available. It is time-consuming to change instruments and for this reason some of them are designed to be multipurpose, for example combined diathermy hook, irrigator and sucker. Versions of most of the stapling machines available in open surgery can be used laparoscopically (see Ch. 2). Blood vessels can be isolated and ligated; intraperitoneal ligature tying has largely superseded extraperitoneal knot-tying. Sutures and suture ligatures are similarly inserted and tied intraperitoneally. Clips can be applied and an intraperitoneal stapling machine, resembling a miniature GIA intestinal stapler, safely inserts lines of staples on each side as it divides larger vessels or ducts.

6. Dissection techniques have been modified from those used in open surgery. Wherever possible the tissues are separated into layers and sequentially identified and sealed. Unipolar diathermy has long been a popular and effective method; small amounts of tissue are separated, hooked up clear of the main mass, identified, coagulated and simultaneously divided. Bipolar diathermy is increasingly popular. Because your view is restricted, you may not notice that tissue outside the intended area has been burned via metal in contact with the diathermy applicator. When two metal instruments are in close proximity and the alternating diathermy current is passed through one, it may induce a current in the other, even though they are insulated from each other, and so the current may reach the patient. Use the lowest

power setting, prefer bipolar to monopolar and select cutting in preference to coagulation current.

7. Vessels can also be sealed after clamping to appose the walls using electrosurgery, with the Ligasure™ system which automatically senses the melting of collagen to weld the walls. The harmonic scalpel ultrasonic coagulator and cutting device coapts and seals the tissues with a protein coagulum at the relatively low temperature, compared with electrosurgical instruments, of 50–100°C. In some cases large masses are disrupted using laser beams. Dissection through solid tissues using simple or sophisticated instruments demands the greatest familiarity and highest skills – but can be achieved by experts.

8. Because your hands may be widely separated (Fig. 13.5), they cannot be held as steadily as they would be during open surgery when the base can usually be brought close to the point of action, and the hands are close together working in practised harmony.

9. The most experienced assistant takes charge of the camera. Since multiple access ports are used, you can delegate to assistants responsibility for some instruments. Some surgeons use voice directed, body or eye movement directed control, in the absence of an experienced assistant. Retraction and steadying of tissues can be delegated to another; a number of versatile retractors and graspers have been designed.

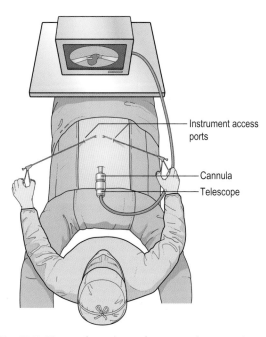

Fig. 13.5 Diagram from above of a surgeon laparotomist manipulating instruments while watching the television monitor connected to the camera inserted into the patient's peritoneal cavity.

Instrument access ports

Cannula

Telescope

10. Excised tissues can sometimes be withdrawn through the largest or a surgically enlarged port site or fresh incision. A useful method is to place the tissue within a strong, flexible bag, bring out the neck of the bag through a small exit hole and exert traction combined with a side-to-side motion to draw it out. Alternatively, a morcellator (F *morceau*, cognate with morsel, from L *mordere* = to bite) can be used to chop up a large piece of tissue into small particles within the bag for withdrawal through a small exit port. In women you can create a posterior colpotomy (G *kolpos* = vagina).

11. A variety of procedures are 'laparoscopy assisted', part open surgery, part laparoscopy. In some cases dissection is performed laparoscopically and anastomoses are fashioned at the surface. In low rectal anastomoses, circular staplers can be inserted trans-anally. Hand assistance can be employed using a special glove sealed to the margins of an incision. Although such procedures may take longer than purely open operations they often cause less disturbance and recovery is quicker.

CLOSURE

1. At the end of the procedure, first carefully check that there has been no inadvertent damage, no residual bleeding, and no free bodies left in the peritoneal cavity.

2. Remove each instrument in turn while observing the withdrawal from within, to guard against herniation into the defects.

3. Close each secondary port hole after ensuring that there is no bleeding within the track. Inject bupivacaine into the surrounding tissues and close the fascia using interrupted stitches. Insert a single subcuticular synthetic absorbable stitch, then close the skin with adhesive strips.

4. Finally withdraw the laparoscope under vision.

5. Gently compress the abdomen to expel any residual gas.

6. Elevate the margins of the telescope portal by means of the stitches inserted at the beginning of the procedure, and tie them after ensuring that no abdominal contents have insinuated themselves into the gap. Close the skin with adhesive tape.

ACQUIRING SKILLS

1. You need new skills for minimal access procedures beyond those you have acquired for open surgery. Some surgeons find it difficult to adapt.

2. On a flat, two-dimensional screen, you can see the tips of the instruments in relation to the tissues from one aspect only. Misperception from the restricted

view, added to lack of touch sense, leads to incorrect speculative and occasionally wrong conclusions, particularly noted during cholecystectomy,[1] leading to error.

3. In open surgery your hands are close to the point of action of the instruments and are able to feel and assess the tissues, approaching the target from different angles. Now they are at the ends of long shafts, and may be wide apart and well away from the 'business' ends. Coordination of hand movements is difficult to achieve in this unnatural posture and with a limited range of approach to the target. Hand movements do not correspond to those of the instrument tips, being spatially reversed and varying with the relation of the instrument shafts to the abdominal wall, which acts as a fulcrum; novices are found to exert 130–138% greater force and torque than experts to achieve the same result.[2]

4. Minimal access surgery lends itself to material simulation and virtual reality courses more than almost any other formally taught surgical skill. The reason is that you need to learn and practise using a new set of instruments while seeing your objective on a flat screen. It is remarkable how rapidly some surgeons have adapted to the new circumstances by assiduous practice.

Key points

- Remember, though, that the instruments that you learn to wield skilfully are merely intermediaries between you and the living tissues when you come to apply your training to clinical use.
- No simulator has yet been invented that challenges you with living, often diseased, displaced, tissues – the real target of your skills.

5. Every laparoscopic unit should have simulators where trainees can spend spare time acquiring facility with the techniques. This is not yet provided universally and the simulator may not be available when you wish to practise. You can provide yourself with a simple simulator, using cleaned, worn-out or disposable instruments (Fig. 13.6). Start by placing objects in an open-topped box with direct viewing and holding the instruments directly, then introduce them through holes in the lid, and finally cover the top to prevent you from seeing the objects directly by using two mirrors. Practise holding a structure with forceps held in one hand after manipulating it to present it most advantageously, and cutting it with scissors held in the other hand (Fig. 13.7). Practise dissection using, for example, a chicken leg.

6. Suturing is commonly performed in a similar manner to that used in open surgery. In order to facilitate inserting stitches, try to insert them from

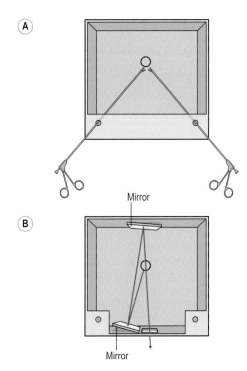

Fig. 13.6 Simple 'home-made' boxes with which to practise minimal access surgery. **A** Remove part of the lid so that you can view the target and instrument tips directly. **B** Place two mirrors so that you can view the target area indirectly. Place a screen so that you cannot see the target directly.

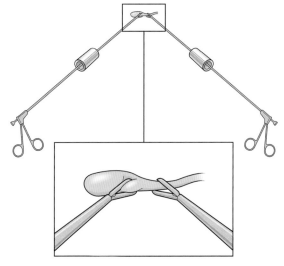

Fig. 13.7 Hold a structure steady using forceps held in one hand while cutting it using scissors held in the other hand.

the dominant to the non-dominant side (Fig 13.8) or from far to near. Make use of your ability to pronate and supinate, to drive the curved needle smoothly through the tissues.

Fig. 13.8 One simple method of intracorporeal suturing. Try to suture from your dominant to non-dominant side, exerting counter pressure on the non-dominant side and steadying the emerging needle to be recaptured and withdrawn with the needle driver.

Fig. 13.10 Roeder preformed knot. The standing part is led to the exterior within a hollow pusher tube. Place the loop over the structure to be ligated. Tighten it by pushing the knot down with the pusher tube against the counter tension on the standing part. The knot will not slip. Cut off the standing part and withdraw it with the pusher tube.

using straight forceps, then with laparoscopy instruments under direct vision, and finally by indirect viewing. Remember that grasping threads with metal instruments severely weakens them, so hold them in parts that will be discarded.

8. Thread ligation and suturing has been greatly reduced by the introduction of mechanical staplers and stapling instruments developed as miniaturized open surgery instruments.

9. Dissection techniques have been modified or adapted. Blunt dissection can be performed using retractors to steady the tissues and against which to create mild tension. Sharp dissection requires preliminary exploration behind the area to exclude vital structures that in open techniques could be palpated or transilluminated from behind. Distension of tissues by injecting saline is an aid to dissection by separating structures. Monopolar diathermy can be applied using a hook to seal, then disrupt flimsy connective tissue, but it can produce smoke that temporarily reduces visibility. Bipolar forceps develop heating only between the tips of the forceps. For piercing and disrupting certain dense tumours, Nd:YAG lasers are sometimes valuable. Ultrasound at a vibration rate of 55 000 cycles/second using a Harmonic scalpel™ is popular because it causes limited heating and does not produce smoke. Because even a slight amount of bleeding obscures the view through the laparoscope, there is an imperative to seal even small blood vessels before dividing them.

Fig. 13.9 Form a half-hitch outside the abdomen and thread one end through the pusher tube. Tighten the half-hitch by pushing down the pusher tube against counter tension exerted on the other thread. Repeat this for the other half-hitch to form a knot.

7. Initially, many knots were created externally and pushed down with a pusher (Fig. 13.9). Pre-knotted loops are available which can be tightened using a pusher, or you may yourself create a Roeder knot (Fig. 13.10). Many laparoscopic surgeons now tie intracorporeal (intraperitoneal) knots constructed in a similar manner to the instrument ties employed in open operations. A simple method is shown step by step in Fig. 13.11 but there are many variations. Initially practise this tie with multifilament threads,

Fig. 13.11 Internal knot-tying resembles the instrument tie described in Chapter 3. **A** The short end is on the right, the long, needled end, is on the left. Slackly raise the left thread with the right forceps and push the thread into a bight with the left forceps. **B** Now pass the left forceps behind the lower part of the bight, **C** in front of the upper part. **D** Draw the right forceps down to keep the thread loop round the left forceps with which now grasp the tip of the short thread on the right. **E** Pull the short thread through the looped long thread and tighten the half-hitch by separating the forceps. **F** Tie the second half-hitch by lifting the long thread slackly with the right forceps while forming a bight by pushing the slack thread to the right with the right forceps. **G** Now pass the right forceps behind the lower part of the bight. **H** Push the tip of the right forceps up in front of the upper bight, **I** while drawing the long thread towards you to keep the loop round the right forceps with which you grasp the short thread. **J** Draw the short end through the loop to form the second half-hitch and tighten it onto the first by separating the forceps.

Key points

- Laparoscopic surgery offers a valuable lesson to general surgeons – haemostasis before dissection.
- Transfer the attitude to open surgery by identifying and sealing blood vessels before, not after, dividing them whenever possible.

Other procedures

1. Because of the pioneering work of Kurt Semm of Kiel in Germany, gynaecologists utilized minimal access techniques before general and other surgeons and have extended the number of procedures that can be carried out by the technique. Large excised structures are frequently removed through the vagina.
2. Urologists pioneered many single channel techniques because of the early development of the cystoscope and have adopted minimal access procedures. Although many of them are endoscopic, it is possible to approach the kidney extraperitoneally, first creating a space by inserting and inflating a balloon without transgressing the peritoneum.
3. Orthopaedic surgeons face the problem that joint spaces are difficult to develop although the supra-patellar pouch of the knee forms a capacious space. Joint spaces are distended not with carbon dioxide but with saline. Arthroscopy often needs to be carried out using general anaesthesia because it is usually necessary to manipulate and distract the joint. Many conditions previously treated by open operation can now be treated in part or whole through minimal access procedures. A torn knee cartilage can be repaired, trimmed, smoothed, reattached, avoiding meniscectomy. Arthroscopic assisted repair of a ruptured anterior cruciate ligament is frequently employed.
4. Thoracoscopic access allows diagnostic inspection and a number of procedures to be performed, including sympathectomy. Cardiovascular surgeons employ minimal access techniques including valve repairs. Cardiac valve replacement can be carried out robotically.
5. Otolaryngologists have pioneered many techniques to provide access to small areas difficult to approach. Operations upon the middle ear and the minute ossicles are now commonplace. Cochlear implants for the relief of deafness are constantly improving.
6. The size of corneo-scleral incisions in ophthalmology was previously large enough to extract a hard, opaque lens. By liquefying the lens using ultrasound phaco-emulsification (G *phakos* = lens) it can then be aspirated and replaced with a soft plastic lens that is rolled up and spontaneously unrolls within the intraocular capsule. This can be carried out through a very small incision.
7. Neurosurgeons have also embraced minimal access techniques in many areas. Localized lesions may be dealt with using stereotactic procedures (G *stereos* = solid + *tassein* = to arrange), first used in 1906 by Robert Clarke and Sir Victor Horsley (1857–1916). The original metal helmet frame is mostly replaced now by three-dimensional computing, allowing electrodes to be inserted through burr holes, for electrical stimulation, DC tissue destruction, or AC coagulation, or to obtain biopsies. Cobalt-60 'gamma-knife' irradiation can be accurately targeted from a specialized helmet after obtaining the three-dimensional coordinates.

REFERENCES

1. Way L, Stewart L, Gantert W, et al. Causes and prevention of laparoscopic bile duct injuries: analysis of 252 cases from a human factors and cognitive psychology perspective. *Ann Surg.* 2003;237:460–469.
2. Rosen J, MacFarlane M, Richards C, et al. Surgeon-tool force/torque signatures: evaluation of surgical skills in minimally invasive surgery. In: *Proceedings of Medicine Meets Virtual Reality, MMVR – 7.* San Francisco, CA: IOS Press; 1999. Online. Available: http://bionics.soe.ucsc.edu/publications/CP_03.pdf June 26, 2009.

Chapter | **14** |

Handling craft skills

Insulted to be referred to as a craftsman? Don't be. In the Middle Ages, surgeons were trained not in universities but as apprentices to Masters. Within a craft a Master can *show* you the required skills, whereas a trainer or coach can teach and correct you but does not necessarily have exceptional skills. The title, shortened to Mr, is proudly retained within Britain and some countries with cultural ties to Britain. Of course, we are physicians first but with the added ability to perform operations.

The surgical craftsman's material is living human flesh. Never forget that all your skill must be targeted at the correct treatment of the tissues; you acquired skill with the instruments to enable you to focus on that commitment. This aim was immortalized by the French surgeon Ambroise Paré (1510–1590), who had the humility to state, 'Je le pansai, Dieu le guérit.' 'I dressed him, God healed him.' Whatever your philosophical beliefs, we cannot *heal* but we owe it to the tissues to help them to heal.

Always keep in mind the precepts associated with Kocher and Halsted. They promoted the importance of careful, gentle surgery, perfect haemostasis and perfect apposition of the tissues. Notice that speed is not included. These concerns remain unaltered, although they are sometimes forgotten or ignored – and I guiltily remember failing to observe them on occasion, resulting in remorseful nights lying awake.

> **Key point**
>
> - Techniques advance but the fundamental precepts of good surgery remain.

PHYSICIAN/SURGEON

1. Never forget that you are primarily a physician with an extra practical skill. Superlative technique on its own is useless. It must be applied correctly at the right time on the right patient. Many surgeons are capable of performing a wide variety of operations but not necessarily of selecting and preparing the patients on whom to perform. Read standard operative texts which describe in detail the individual considerations required for each patient and each procedure. Ensure, for example, that you can justify your decision to recommend the procedure to your patient and that you have

taken every necessary step to ensure that the patient is in the best possible condition, the timing and facilities are correct, operation site marked if appropriate, the informed consent form is signed, suitable prophylaxis is arranged for bleeding, clotting and infective complications, and universal precautions are observed.

2. Keep up to date. Do not become an expert in outdated treatments. Remember, though, that innovators are biased. Their reported good results may stem in part from the selection of patients, perhaps the closer monitoring and care of the patients, and over-optimistic interpretation of the outcomes. Veer towards waiting for reports from surgeons who do not have a personal commitment to the treatment. Remember that in prospective trials it is often necessary to exclude patients in order to keep the number of variables to a minimum. Our methods of audit do not yet fully include and compare those patients who are treated conservatively or by alternative methods.

3. Before the anaesthetic is administered make sure that this is the correct patient and reassure yourself that you are operating on the correct side if this is a unilateral lesion.

4. Do not become a skilful operator who lacks judgement. You may become skilled in a particular technique but others emerge that are shown to produce better results. Be willing to acquire the new skills required rather than continue with an outdated method because you can perform it expertly. The American novelist Mark Twain aptly summed up this attitude with the statement, 'If your only tool is a hammer, every problem begins to look like a nail.' In contrast, if you can produce results at least as good as those obtained by a newer method, you may be wise not to change.

5. There have been remarkable advances in non-surgical treatment of many conditions traditionally treated surgically, including medical treatment, endoscopy and interventional radiology. When you are convinced of their effectiveness, relinquish your patients to those who are expert in the alternative treatment.

6. You rely upon your colleagues in the operating theatre to help you and also to warn you of impending or actual danger or disaster. Maintain an atmosphere in which all feel able to speak out in such circumstance. When you are in doubt, explaining the problem to them often clarifies your course of action, or someone will contribute a valuable suggestion.

Key points

a. A good surgeon knows how to operate.
b. A better surgeon knows when to operate.
c. The best surgeon knows when not to operate.

SKILLS COURSES

1. Quite rightly, trainee surgeons are introduced to operating in courses, with simulations and virtual reality trainers. These allow aspiring operators to familiarize themselves with the procedures and practise using the instruments and equipment. You must acquire familiarity with the instruments so that you can manipulate them skilfully while your primary awareness is directed to the tissues on which you are operating.[1] This applies particularly in minimal access techniques when the movement of the tip is the opposite of handle movement.

2. When you attend a course and are shown how to carry out a procedure it does not transfer a skill to you. It shows you how to perform, but to do so skilfully demands intelligent, assiduous practice.

3. At the end of the course, when you are assessed, the examiner has a list of objectively assessable actions to mark. If you succeed in passing all the steps you pass the assessment. It is a minimum achievement, not a measure of your skill.

4. This is not to decry such courses; they demonstrate many fundamentals, introduce concepts of 'best practice', identify errors early before they become habits. But there are other contributions to successful performance that are not identifiable within the limits of artificiality, time, facilities and limited observation. Success on a course does not signify surgical competence; it attests to correct performance in a number of formalized steps.

Key points

- The gap between learning to manipulate instruments and simulations on courses, and mastery as a surgeon, is between handling the instruments and operating skilfully on live people.
- It is a large, extensible gap, not yet amenable to objective analysis.

5. As in every other complex task, you may observe all the instructions but fail to perform successful surgical operations. The reason is that outcome depends on your ability to assemble the components in the correct sequence and perform each one perfectly for the right indications. This relationship was recognized in the late nineteenth century by the German Gestalt psychologists (Ger *gestellt* = put together): '*The whole is greater than the sum of the parts.*' The purpose of this chapter is to emphasize how you must combine your individual aptitudes to create a fully competent surgeon.

OPERATING PRECEPTS

Gentleness

Living tissues are easily damaged by rough handling. If previously normal tissues are traumatized they usually survive. The vitality of already traumatized or diseased tissues is already prejudiced.

1. Rough handing does not show up now but healing will be delayed or fail, and resistance to infection is lowered. Gentle handling has to be a one hundred per cent habit. Never grasp tissue with a metal instrument to displace it, when it can be gently manipulated with a finger, swab, encircling thread or tube, retractor or a closed forceps.
2. If you crush tissue and release it, within a few moments the vessels will fill with blood and it will look normal; but it is not normal. It will die in part or whole. If it survives, healing will be delayed, dead or dying cells will be replaced by scar tissue and if the scar is subjected to tension it will become stretched. When incisions have been closed with stitches that are too tight, they produce wound scars showing a ladder pattern of white scars resulting from the death of tissue strangled within the stitches.
3. Over-distension of closed spaces and vessels is a frequently overlooked form of trauma. Muscular walls are overstretched and temporarily paralysed or torn and will give way. The delicate cellular lining of overfilled vessels is disrupted, exposing the basement membrane. If such a vessel is united to another, the integrity of the union is prejudiced. In the case of blood vessels, platelets adhere to the bared subintima as a basis for clots that may block the lumen. When mobilizing structures, beware of forcefully stripping them. Veins mobilized for arterial bypass undergo spasm if the adventitia is stripped off.[2]

'Setting up'

This aspect of operating is not well recognized but is in fact vitally important. Watch an expert craftsman in any occupation and you will notice how slowly and carefully the preliminaries are carried out, the problem examined and assessed, the equipment assembled, checked and laid out, the planning of the approach. When the procedure is finally undertaken it proceeds smoothly and faultlessly.

1. In the past, when surgeons worked with relatively stable teams, they could rely with confidence on preparedness and checks, even though they knew that the ultimate responsibility was theirs.
2. You may not work in an established, stable team. Ensure that you personally check the full list of requirements, or are assured by someone in whom you have complete trust.
3. Do not start until you have personally checked that everything you need is available, is working, and if it is something that is likely to fail, you have a functioning back-up.
4. As you start the operation, if there is anything that could possibly complicate the operation or make it more difficult, correct it now.
5. If you are carrying out a manoeuvre that feels unnatural, stop and consider approaching it from another aspect, perhaps by changing your approach or moving to the other side of the operating table.

Key points

- When you are delegated a task, do not rush to 'get on with it'.
- Carefully assess what needs to be done, identify what you need and how you should carry it out.
- Start cautiously. Make all your movements carefully and slowly.
- Nothing makes the person who delegated the task more apprehensive than watching you rush headlong into the risk of a disaster.

Speed

Obsession with speed is one of the most dangerous and damaging characteristics. It is often driven by the unintelligent belief that by completing an operation at breakneck speed the operator is demonstrating his or her expertise. William, one of the famous Mayo brothers of Rochester, is reported to have left an operation being performed by William Halsted after three hours, muttering sarcastically, 'That's the first time I have seen the top end of the wound healing, while the bottom end is still being operated on.' Time has proved Halsted right.

1. You should have understood, before you entered the operating theatre, that when you have acquired a skill in performing a particular procedure you must perform it at a natural pace; otherwise what is ideally accomplished automatically and perfectly is raised to conscious focus and so is performed clumsily.
2. Hand speed and operating speed are different. Performing an action in a hurry very often fails, requiring to be repeated, so that the total time taken is the same as if it were performed at a natural speed. What is wasteful of time is unnecessary and ineffectual actions, often from lack of certainty regarding the correct next step.

Key point

- Next time you are uncertain, stop moving and devote your energies to making the correct decision.

Sequence

1. Unless there are special circumstances, employ the standard sequences that have been developed over many years. If you do not, you may discover that you have prejudiced your access to an important area, inadvertently damaged an important structure or prejudiced local function.
2. Operate deliberately and naturally.
3. As a rule, complete and check each step of the operation before proceeding to the next.

Strategy/tactics

1. These terms, which are often confused, are important concepts if you wish to be a successful surgeon.
2. Strategy (G *stratos* = an army + *agein* = to lead: generalship). Your planning and preparation of yourself, your patient, team, equipment and back-up are essential. Consider what you will do if there are unexpected findings or complications – often called, 'what if's'.
3. Tactics (G *tassein* = to arrange; was applied to manoeuvring in the presence of the enemy). It refers to how you react to what happens during the operation; how you identify, interpret, avoid and respond to unforeseen problems. For many circumstances, guidelines are laid down and usually you should adhere to them but exceptionally you recognize that the problem does not conform to that described in the guidelines.

Key points

- Do not dismiss an unusual finding. Investigate it and interpret it.
- Do not rigidly continue the intended actions if the new finding makes them inappropriate.
- Carefully assess your competence to deal with the new situation and react accordingly.

Tissue oxygenation

1. Kocher and Halsted did not have access to methods of determining tissue oxygenation. They, and many of their successors, could determine vitality only by arterial pulsation and colour.
2. We now have methods of determining the oxygen concentration. An important contribution was made by Tom Hunt of San Francisco, who measured the concentration of interstitial oxygen concentration in closed wounds and found that it is severely reduced, especially immediately after operation, and this is often not clinically evident.[3] In contrast, when the method of delayed primary closure is employed, the wound tissues are in contact with atmospheric oxygen concentrations.
3. Hypoxic tissues are particularly susceptible to infection with anaerobic or micro-aerophilic organisms. In case of doubt, delayed primary closure

of wounds ensures that tissues are in contact with oxygen at atmospheric pressure.

EMERGENCIES

'Emergency' (from 'emerge', L *e* = out of + *mergere* = to plunge; to arise out of) suggests an unexpected occurrence requiring immediate action. What is often left out is the importance of recognizing exactly what has happened, what it means and what is the best way of dealing with it. Unintelligent action often makes matters worse.

1. If something unexpected happens during an operation, *assess it*. Do nothing until you have done so.
2. For many emergency situations, studies have produced guidelines that are suitable for most circumstances. Learn them. Practise the prescribed actions.
3. *Bleeding* is a common emergency. Very often, simple finger pressure is the best immediate action and rushing to apply metal haemostats may be a disaster.
4. *Over-reaction* often extends to performing unnecessary procedures as a guard against possible complications.
5. Once you have dealt with the emergency, check that you have not caused or missed further damage.
6. Check that you have achieved your objective and then close.

Key points

- Do not lightly abandon safe routines in an emergency.
- Perform the simplest procedure that corrects the emergency situation – and nothing more.

ERROR AVOIDANCE

You are in a high-risk profession. You will make misjudgements and technical errors.

Key points

- If you embark on an operation without first acquiring or revising the anatomy, you are inviting disaster.
- Missiles, spreading infections, malignant tumours are not respecters of tissue planes or anatomical boundaries.

---

1. Many surgical errors occur before the patient reaches the operating theatre, in the selection and preparation of patients, operations and numerous requirements of equipment, back-up and technical support. Further errors occur following operation as a result of inadequate monitoring and failure to respond effectively to deterioration.

2. Accept that we are all fallible. Any surgeon who claims not to have made any mistakes is either inexperienced, suffering from self-delusion or is a liar. Those who are concerned with organizations requiring high reliability try to identify changes to the system incorporating safeguards. Procedural rules and guidelines incorporate practice that has been shown to be safest overall. Remember, though, that when planning an investigation, in order to reduce the number of variables, some combinations are excluded from the trials. You may in clinical practice encounter such circumstances where the guidelines do not apply. You must recognize this and ask for advice and help.

3. Whereas it is traditional to try to eliminate human variability, it is now recognized that human compensatory and adaptive responses to changing events represent an important safeguard. It is this very variability and adaptability of humans' dynamic reactions to rare but dangerous events that can be drawn upon.[4]

4. As a trainee, if you encounter an unusual situation seeming to require exceptional management, do not implement your intentions before discussing it with a senior colleague. Often, what is new to you is well known to experienced colleagues, who are also aware of the risks.

5. Errors at operation may be the result of lack of skilful performance such as overuse of force, coincident damage to nearby structures and clumsily performed procedures. It is far more likely that you make an error of judgement.

6. Do not be misguided enough to believe that since it is your error, you are honour-bound to repair it. As a trainee be humble enough to recognize that recovering the situation is best carried out by an expert.

Key points

- If you damage an important structure, the most crucial actions are to recognize it and react to it.
- Most such damage is best dealt with now.
- Ask yourself, 'Am I competent to deal with it or should I call for help?'

7. A much more frequent cause of error, especially in minimal access operations but also occurring in open operations, is *misperception*. Once a mistaken assumption is made about the nature of a structure, it is likely to persist and you may accommodate subsequent findings around it. A notorious mistake when operating on an infantile inguinal hernia is to mistake the thickened (Scarpa's) deep fascia for the external oblique aponeurosis. As a result of the misperception, you may not identify the external inguinal ring.

8. In open operations you run doubtful structures between your fingers to trace them, feel the texture

and mobility. During a minimal access procedure you are deprived of haptic input – the sensation of touch, to note the surface and temperature, consistency and kinaesthetic (G *kinein* = to move + *aisthesis* = perception) appreciation of contours and attachments. As a result, serious ductal injuries occur more frequently than during open operations.[5]

9. Some people who appear to be concentrating seem not to anticipate imminent accidents although these are evident to onlookers. When the error is perpetrated the surgeon expresses surprise as though it was a unique occurrence.

Key points

- If you have limited access to confirm your first impression, do not proceed.
- Doubly check it; trace the limits of an identified structure to confirm its nature.

ASSISTING AT OPERATIONS

1. Do not spurn the opportunity to assist. You will learn how to do it – and sometimes, how not to do it. It is also your opportunity to demonstrate your assiduous attention and trustworthiness that encourages the surgeon to delegate part or all of the procedure to you, under expert guidance, admonishment and encouragement.

2. Do not look upon assisting as a necessary boring prelude to carrying out the procedure yourself. The privilege of assisting a skilled operator allows you to acquire judgement and technique both consciously and unconsciously, so that when you come to perform the procedure yourself, you will automatically adopt safe and effective techniques.

3. Read up the anatomy and pathology that will be important, the night before. This will enormously increase the value you will gain from assisting at the operation.

4. Observe every manoeuvre and at opportune moments enquire if you do not understand the reason for it.

5. Note that the surgeon performs some manoeuvres in a routine, relaxed fashion, while taking extreme care over other parts. Make sure you know why.

6. Notice that good surgeons keep the operative field tidy.

7. As you are asked to assist, try to anticipate what is required without seeming to try and take over the operation. If you are asked your opinion, give it quietly and honestly. If you think you have seen something the surgeon has missed or you think a mistake is about to be made, say so. If your warning

has been heard but there is no change of the action, recognize that it is the surgeon's responsibility. Afterwards, at an opportune moment, discuss the matter to improve your understanding.

8. Do not be dazzled by technical brilliance while being, as yet, unaware of the more important judgements that have to be made. They are rarely black and white – more usually they are shades of grey – and the particular shade is contentious.

9. If you are fortunate enough to be delegated part of the operation, concentrate on being calm and careful.

10. As you become more competent and are given more personal responsibility you will learn even more from assisting than formerly, since you are then more aware of the problems. You may then be awarded the privileged relationship with the surgeon of being treated on equal terms while you both discuss and demonstrate the finer points of operative surgery.

11. Later in your career you may be privileged to assist your own trainees. It is not a one-way teaching experience. My own career has been nourished and made enjoyable, by a series of outstanding, expert, assiduous, supportive and trustworthy junior colleagues.

MENTORING

1. In the past it was an accepted, informal practice for surgeons at all stages of their careers to attend operations carried out by recognized experts, and they were frequently invited to 'scrub up' and assist, in some cases, even having parts of the operation delegated to them. It was possible to watch many senior colleagues and pick up a great deal of knowledge both consciously and by unconscious 'osmosis'. This valuable facility is no longer possible.

2. Modern surgeons are able to apply for consultant posts when they have much less experience than their predecessors. Many acknowledge this and avoid taking on difficult procedures that are at the limit of their competence. As always happens in progressive societies, surgeons have adapted by seeking further training in their deficient areas.

3. In many specialties the system of mentoring is already in place. A surgeon wishing to take on a new procedure attends formal courses and then joins an experienced surgeon as an assistant, then a monitored operator until the senior surgeon is able to declare the trainee as competent. When the competent but still inexperienced surgeon is authorized to perform unsupervised, the outcomes are carefully audited to ensure that the results are satisfactory.

4. Do not ever fail to accept assistance from a more experienced colleague, even though you may feel fully competent and experienced. I have found it a two-way learning experience.

Ten reminders

- Operative skill alone does not guarantee surgical success. It is one component, albeit vital, of your general care of the patient as a medical practitioner.
- Do not try to be a skilful surgeon only when you are in the operating theatre. Make it part of your normal behaviour to perform everyday practical tasks neatly, smoothly, with minimal force (see Ch. 1).
- Resist the temptation to 'get on with it'. Double check that you have tested equipment and instruments within easy reach, and that the field is otherwise clear of unnecessary – and especially loose – objects. Are you approaching the task in the most natural relationship?
- As a craftsman whose material is living tissue, never turn aside from an opportunity to examine it, study its anatomical relationships and assess its physical properties. Remember that diseases and missiles are not respecters of anatomical boundaries.
- Because you use instruments as intermediaries, practise using them in simulators, virtual reality trainers, skills courses and on simple home-made mock-ups until you do not have to think about them and can concentrate on what is happening at the real target of your skill – human flesh.
- Watch experts. You acquire knowledge consciously by noting how they tackle problems and you will acquire knowledge unconsciously – the type of knowledge that is not easy to put into words.
- Prepare for and react to unexpected findings. Do not insist on pursuing your original intention but reassess it.
- Do not try to hurry. Your concentration switches from the overall objective to the activities that are normally performed with your subsidiary awareness.
- Do not forget the vital factor of tissue oxygenation. Phagocytes deprived of it are inactivated, making the tissues susceptible to infection, and prejudicing healing.
- A major operation is merely a series of minor procedures; but for success, every small step must be perfect.

COMMON SENSE

With the intention of preventing people from making stupid errors, experts are from time to time asked to draw up guidelines. These cannot cover every eventuality but are intended to give the greatest protection to the majority of people at risk. Use them but be aware of exceptional circumstances where they do not apply. This common sense attitude was exemplified by the famous, legless British fighter pilot ace, Sir Douglas Bader (1910–1982), 'Rules are for the guidance of wise men and the blind obedience of fools.'

REFERENCES

1. Polanyi M. *Personal knowledge*. London: Routledge and Kegan Paul; 1973.

2. Loesch A, Dashwood MR, Souza DSR. Does the method of harvesting the saphenous vein for coronary artery bypass surgery affect venous smooth muscle cells? iNOS immunolabelling and ultrastructural findings. *International Journal of Surgery*. 2006;4:20–29.

3. Chang N, Goodson 3rd WH, Gottrup F, Hunt TK. Direct measurement of wound and tissue oxygen tension in postoperative patients. *Ann Surg*. 1983;197:470–478.

4. Reason J. Human error: models and management. *BMJ*. 2008;320:768–770.

5. Way L, Stewart L, Gantert W, et al. Causes and prevention of laparoscopic bile duct injuries: analysis of 252 cases from a human factors and cognitive psychology perspective. *Ann Surg*. 2003;237:450–469.

Index

Index

Index